D0053822

your child's teeth

617.6 STE
Sterling, Evelina Weidman, 1970-
Your child's teeth

YOUR CHILD'S
TEETH

A Complete Guide for Parents

EVELINA WEIDMAN STERLING

and **ANGIE BEST-BOSS**

DISCARD

The Johns Hopkins University Press
BALTIMORE

PARK CITY LIBRARY
1255 Park Avenue
P.O. Box 668
Park City, Utah 84060
Phone: (435) 615-5600

NOTE TO READER: This book describes how to protect the dental health of children *in general*. It was not written about *your* child. The services of a competent dental or medical professional should be obtained whenever medical or other specific advice is needed.

© 2013 The Johns Hopkins University Press
All rights reserved. Published 2013
Printed in the United States of America on
acid-free paper
9 8 7 6 5 4 3 2 1

The Johns Hopkins University Press
2715 North Charles Street
Baltimore, Maryland 21218-4363
www.press.jhu.edu

*Special discounts are available for bulk pur-
chases of this book. For more information,
please contact Special Sales at 410-516-6936 or
specialsales@press.jhu.edu.*

The Johns Hopkins University Press uses envi-
ronmentally friendly book materials, including
recycled text paper that is composed of at least
30 percent post-consumer waste, whenever
possible.

LIBRARY OF CONGRESS
CATALOGING-IN-PUBLICATION DATA

Sterling, Evelina Weidman, 1970–
Your child's teeth : a complete guide for parents
/ Evelina Weidman Sterling, Angie Best-Boss.
    pages   cm
  Includes index.
  ISBN-13: 978-1-4214-1062-3 (hardcover : alk.
paper)
  ISBN-10: 1-4214-1062-1 (hardcover : alk.
paper)
  ISBN-13: 978-1-4214-1063-0 (pbk. : alk. paper)
  ISBN-10: 1-4214-1063-X (pbk. : alk. paper)
[etc.]
  1. Children—Dental care. 2. Pedodontics.
I. Best-Boss, Angie. II. Title.
  RK55.C5S74 2013
  617.6'45—dc23   2012047776

A catalog record for this book is available from
the British Library.

CONTENTS

FOREWORD

As a mother and a grandmother, I find nothing more precious than the smile of a child. A child's smile can warm your heart on the coldest day and bring joy to all who experience it. As president and CFO of National Children's Oral Health Foundation: *America's ToothFairy*, I have witnessed the devastating effects that poor oral health has on our children, our communities, and our future.

Your Child's Teeth: A Complete Guide for Parents provides parents and caregivers a clear understanding of how oral health is inextricably linked to overall systemic health, because the mouth is the gateway to the body. Covering everything, including basic preventive strategies, nutrition, oral care for a child with special needs, and various dental problems and treatments for children of all ages, the book is a comprehensive guide on how to make sure your child maintains good oral health for a lifetime. *America's ToothFairy* and our pediatric dental experts are proud to have been collaborators from the inception of this book. This important project perfectly aligns with our mission of eliminating children's pain and suffering caused by the number one chronic childhood disease in America: preventable tooth decay.

Pediatric dental disease has reached epidemic proportions. Every child deserves a healthy smile, yet millions of children suffer tremendous pain and embarrassment from dental disease, more commonly known as severe tooth decay. Covering their smiles and unable to eat, sleep, or concentrate in school, children with dental disease find themselves in a downward spiral that negatively affects their adult lives. With limited or no access to oral health care, disadvantaged children are at great risk for impaired cognitive and social development, educational disparities, and a lifetime of pain and shame associated with tooth decay.

Oral health education is the key to breaking the cycle of pediatric dental disease. We are grateful to Evelina Weidman Sterling and Angie Best-Boss for their vision and commitment in developing this important health resource for parents and caregivers. This book should be part of every family's library and a vital resource in every child health and welfare institution. By promoting positive oral health behaviors and implementing preventive strategies, we can help make sure that all children have the building blocks they need for happy, healthy futures.

FERN INGBER, M.ED.
President and CEO
National Children's Oral Health Foundation: *America's ToothFairy*

PREFACE

For over two decades now, we have both been fortunate to participate in various aspects of educating patients about important health issues. Imagine our surprise when we tried to find comprehensive and reliable information whenever one of our children had a dental issue and found almost nothing. We decided to use our skills in health education to change this. We envisioned writing a resource similar to the plethora of pediatric health books available today that families would be able to keep on hand and turn to whenever they had a question or concern (big or small) about their children's teeth.

We want to thank the many people who helped make this book possible. We could not have done this without the tremendous support of Fern Ingber, president of the National Children's Oral Health Foundation, also known as America's ToothFairy, as well as the rest of her fabulous staff. Fern connected us with Dr. Martha Ann Keels and Dr. Rebecca Slayton, who graciously shared their expertise about pediatric oral health and were willing to answer all questions we had. We would also like to thank Dr. John H. Taylor, a pediatric dentist practicing in Marietta, Georgia, for giving us invaluable feedback, especially regarding orthodontia, that only someone who genuinely cares about his patients and their families could have provided. Dr. Kenneth A. Murphy of Atlanta, Georgia, was also incredibly helpful as he shared with us the latest and greatest dental technologies. We are especially grateful to our editor, Jackie Wehmueller, for believing in us from the beginning and encouraging us throughout the writing process, and to Melanie Mallon for her editing skills and sharp attention to detail. Finally, we are forever indebted to our families—Dan, Ben, Ellie, DuWain, Kaylyn, Clara, and Katy—for seeing us through yet another book.

Good oral health is a cornerstone for overall health and wellness for everyone. Through this book, we want to share our passion for health and all the knowledge we have gained about children's oral health in order to keep families far and wide smiling brightly for many years to come.

PART I

▼　▼　▼

Introduction

CHAPTER 1

A Guide to Your Child's Teeth

Whether it's your baby's first smile, toddler's toothy grin, or adolescent's shy laughter, you love your child's smile, and you want to do everything you can to protect it. But for a lot of parents, that's easier said than done. A glimpse into most parents' to-do list tells the story. Between helping with homework, making dinner, chauffeuring kids to soccer practice, and other activities, most parents barely have time to brush their children's teeth, much less spend much time thinking about their overall oral health. As a result, most parents encourage their children to brush regularly, get to the dentist when they can, and hope for the best.

Why Good Dental Health Is Important for All Children

Your child's oral health is more important than you may realize. Oral health can offer clues about overall health and wellness. Problems with our mouths can affect the rest of our bodies. Understanding the intimate connection between oral health and general health is enormously helpful when you consider what you can do to protect your child's smile. While it sounds improbable, untreated cavities can lead to painful and some-times even fatal infections. The National Maternal and Child Oral Health Resource Center identifies this and other potential difficulties from neglecting our teeth and oral health:

- Infections from tooth decay or gum disease: as we get older, chronic oral infections can lead to other serious health problems, including heart disease and diabetes
- Difficulty chewing food, which could result in poor nutrition and, in turn, impaired physical development
- Trouble concentrating and learning, as well as absences from school because of pain: according to the *Surgeon General's Report on Oral Health in America* (2000), more than 51 million school hours are lost each year due to dental-related illnesses
- Psychological problems such as low self-esteem and higher risk for social stigma because of decayed teeth and chronic bad breath
- Fewer life opportunities compared to their peers with good oral health

> *Can You Repeat That?*
>
> You may not realize that your child's oral health can affect speech. Having teeth in the right places at the right times helps us speak clearly. For example, the shape of the arch inside the mouth affects how we talk. Many letters of the alphabet cannot be properly pronounced without the help of teeth and bite.

A National Problem

Dental care is the single greatest unmet need for health services among children. More than one in five children—that's 6 million kids—do not receive the care they need every year. Tooth decay is one of the most common childhood diseases, affecting nearly 60 percent of all children. Most of these children come from less financially secure families who face disproportionately high barriers to getting appropriate dental care. For families who struggle financially, paying for preventive dental care, taking time off work for appointments, and even finding a dentist can be difficult. Some parents do not speak English as a first language, which can be an additional obstacle in interacting with health care providers.

More than 50 percent of 6- to 11-year-olds have had cavities or tooth decay in their primary teeth, and nearly 70 percent of 16- to 19-year-olds have had cavities in some permanent teeth. Unfortunately, tooth decay has significantly increased over the past fifteen years. But cavities aren't the only problem that can affect teeth. Children face many threats to a healthy smile, including everything from birth defects and tobacco use to sports injuries and crooked teeth. Keeping their children's teeth clean and healthy can be a challenge for caregivers—especially when those children aren't always willing to cooperate. Many tooth troubles can be prevented, however, and those that can't can usually be treated by experienced dentists.

Your Child's Teeth Inside and Out

Teeth have to be pretty tough to survive a lifetime of chewing, crunching, talking, and the occasional nail biting and soccer ball bump. You may already know that teeth are not primarily made of bone. You may not realize, however, that the part of teeth above the gum line is made of different materials than what's found underneath the gums. Think of your tooth as an iceberg—there's a lot more to it than you can see with your eyes.

> **Your Smile Matters**
>
> Nearly all Americans (99.7 percent, in fact) believe a smile is a valuable social asset. A study from the American Academy of Cosmetic Dentistry (AACD) in 2004 found that 96 percent of adults believe an attractive smile makes a person more appealing and that 74 percent of adults feel an unattractive smile can hurt a person's chances for career success. Do everything you can now to protect your child's smile for social and professional success down the road.

What is the outside of teeth made of?

The part of the tooth that you can see when your child smiles and talks is called a crown. The rounded high parts of the back teeth are cusps. The hard white outer covering of the tooth is the enamel. That thin layer of enamel covers and protects the crown. Tooth enamel is the hardest structure in the human body.

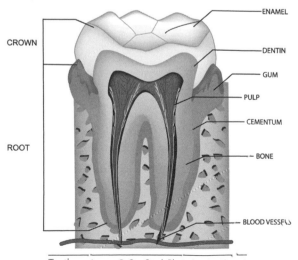

Tooth anatomy. © Can Stock Photo Inc./venimart

What's inside the tooth?

Enamel covers the dentin, which is the second hardest substance in the human body. Dentin makes up most of the tooth and is harder and denser than human bone.

Dentin covers the pulp, which primarily contains blood vessels, nerves, connective tissue, and other components that keep the tooth alive and functional. The pulp supplies your teeth with the nutrients to stay "alive"

How Many Teeth?

A baby's teeth usually begin to come in between 6 and 8 months of age. These teeth are also known as deciduous, primary, or "falling out" teeth. By the age of 30 months, a child usually has a full complement of twenty primary teeth. By age 6, permanent teeth begin to come in. As they grow, they push out the primary teeth, replacing them and filling out the spaces in the jaw.

Adults have thirty-two permanent teeth. Twenty permanent teeth replace the baby teeth that fall out, and another twelve permanent molars will erupt without a primary tooth falling out. Be on the lookout for these molars at around ages 6, 12, and 18. Depending on their age, children may have fewer teeth at any given time because they may lose baby teeth before their adult teeth grow.

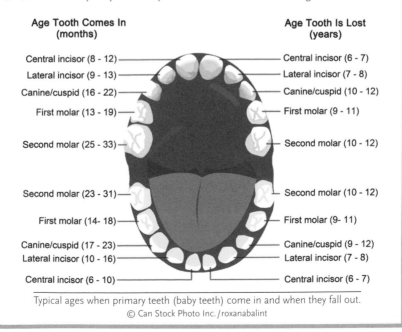

Typical ages when primary teeth (baby teeth) come in and when they fall out.
© Can Stock Photo Inc. / roxanabalint

and in your mouth. The blood vessels and nerves in the pulp enter through the root of the tooth, underneath the gum line.

The root is connected to the tooth above the gum by the neck of the tooth, the part that narrows as it goes into the gum. The root, which lies in a bony socket, makes up about two-thirds of the length of the tooth. It has the same dentin and pulp, but instead of enamel, the root is covered and protected by a thin, bonelike tissue called cementum. This tissue is calcified (made of tough calcium deposits), although it is not as hard as enamel.

Cementum has an important job—it holds the tooth to the surrounding bone. It does this by forming fibers that connect with fibers from the bone socket. Without these fibers, the tooth would not be attached to the jaw bone and would fall out easily.

A tooth is a tooth, right?

Each tooth is different in shape and size. Overall, similar teeth are grouped together depending on their job, such as biting, chewing, or tearing food.

- *Incisors.* These are the eight teeth located in the front of the mouth (four on the top and four on the bottom). Their main job is to cut food, so they are sharp and chisel shaped.
- *Canines.* The four canine teeth (also known as cuspids) are located on either side of the four incisors on top and bottom. Because they are meant to hold and tear food, they have pointed edges.
- *Premolars.* These are the four pairs of teeth located directly next to the canines. Also called bicuspids, their job is to crush and tear food as you eat.
- *Molars.* Molars have wide surfaces for grinding food in the back of the mouth. There are eight molars, in sets of two, on the top and bottom on both sides of the mouth. They usually grow in during middle childhood.

> *Your Teeth*
> *Guide Your Menu*
>
> All our teeth grouped together are called our dentition. The variety of different shapes our teeth come in allows humans to be omnivores. This means we eat both meat and plants. Most animals have more specialized teeth. Meat-eating, or carnivorous, animals like wolves and sharks usually have long, sharp, tearing teeth, and plant-eating animals like cows and horses have large flat teeth for grinding up grass and other vegetation.

• *Third molars.* These four teeth are located in the far back of the mouth—one at each corner. More commonly known as wisdom teeth, they usually do not appear until late teens or adulthood, if at all. Because there may not be enough room for them to erupt, wisdom teeth can become impacted (stuck under gum or bone) and often require surgical removal.

How do I know which tooth the dentist is talking about?

Dentists and dental assistants communicate about specific teeth using a numbering system. Over the years, more than twenty different teeth-numbering systems have been developed, but most general dentists in the United States use the Universal Numbering System. In charts and paperwork, dentists will refer to a particular tooth using the numeric (or, in some cases, alphabetic) notation. You may see the Universal Numbering System used on insurance paperwork, to identify work done on specific teeth.

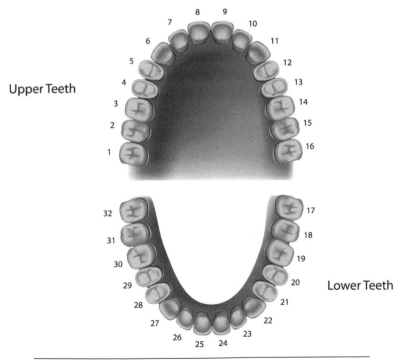

Tooth numbering showing the thirty-two adult teeth. © Can Stock Photo Inc. / alila

A second numbering system, called the Palmer Notation Method, is used by many orthodontists and oral surgeons.

What's the big deal about baby teeth? They're just going to fall out anyway, right?

Unfortunately, many parents think that they don't need to be concerned about baby teeth. It can be tempting to think that only the permanent ones matter. But broken, missing, or cavity-filled baby teeth can lead to a host of serious problems for those permanent teeth waiting in the wings. Baby teeth serve important functions:

- Help children chew healthy foods, therefore providing nutrition
- Help make speech possible
- Aid in the normal development of jaw bones and facial muscles
- Add to an attractive appearance
- Reserve space for the permanent teeth and help guide them into position

While some baby teeth last for only four or five years, those back primary teeth hang in a while longer—sometimes until the child is 11 to 12 years old. If those primary teeth are carrying dental infected and pass that infection on to th that new molar comes in surround long before it is fighting to stay h

If a primary tooth is lost at risk. In fact, sometimes ad make enough space for an une.

When Teeth Go Missing

Hypodontia is the name of a condition in which some of a child's teeth (primary or permanent) never develop—usually up to six teeth, not including wisdom teeth. When more than six teeth are missing, this condition is called oligodontia. In rare cases, all teeth are missing, which is called anodontia. About 30 to 50 percent of people with missing primary teeth have missing permanent teeth as well.

Although the exact cause for missing teeth is unknown, many believe it has to do with genetics (with more females having missing teeth than males or environmental fac that affect tooth opment. It related t nal teeth as just baby teeth; instead start thinking of them as foundational teeth. Healthy primary teeth are the foundation for a healthy set of secondary, or permanent, teeth.

More than Teeth

Poor oral hygiene can cause problems in several different areas of the mouth, but so can sports injuries, trauma, birth defects, nutritional deficiencies, and other illnesses. Parents need to get in the habit of regularly looking inside their child's mouth between dental visits to look for any problems. After all, those pearly whites matter, but they aren't the only parts of your child's mouth that need attention. Your child's oral health involves the structures of the mouth, which include the teeth, gums, palate, tongue, inside of the cheeks, bones and associated muscles, nerves, glands, and blood vessels. During regular visual inspections, be on the lookout for

- broken, cracked, or chipped teeth
- dark spots or holes on surfaces of teeth
- pocked, pitted, or discolored teeth
- sores on the child's gums, tongue, or cheeks
- red, swollen, or puffy gums

If something has changed since the last dental visit, then call your d's dentist and make an appointment.

vill I know if there is a dental problem?

be able to spot a dental problem if your child complains of buble chewing, or if something doesn't look right. Although with visual inspections, early dental problems can be hard ouths. Your child will need regular visits with a dentist healthy teeth but to rule out existing issues. Plus, tooth up in other ways, such as ear pain or headaches, or even in dietary deficiencies when children don't want to eat foods that are difficult to chew. In other words, your child can have dental problems and you could have no idea it's happening.

No child is immune from dental health problems. By the age of 17, one in ten children has already lost at least one permanent tooth to decay. Millions more children are already on the way to a lifetime of poor dental health, increasing their risk of related physical problems. By taking a few specific steps, you can establish a pattern to help ensure that your child, whether in utero or in high school, has a healthy smile for a lifetime. Children's teeth, gums, and tongue are critical to overall health and well-being. In addition to helping with eating and talking, oral health affects many other aspects of life, such as smiling, kissing, singing, playing a musical instrument, smelling and crying. A mouth free of cavities, gum disease, and injury contributes to children's healthy development and success in school and in life.

CHAPTER 2

Basic Care and Cleaning

"This is so cool, Dad. Check it out!" Six-year-old Aaron ran across the kitchen, flashing his toothy grin at his father. After a presentation at school, Aaron had been given plaque-disclosing tablets to use after he brushed his teeth, and although he thought the purple splotches on his teeth were "cool," his father was less impressed. Looking at their sweet smiles, it can be hard to believe just how dirty children's teeth can become.

How dirty can your mouth be? There are literally billions of bacteria (germs) in the mouth covering more than six hundred different species. While any bacteria may seem gross, most are not dangerous. They are found in every mouth, even the cleanest. Saliva helps keep bacteria under control, and stomach enzymes kill those you swallow. Still, good oral hygiene is important because bacteria that build up will cause gum disease and tooth decay.

Why Cleaning Teeth Is Important

One of the most important reasons to clean teeth is to get rid of plaque. Plaque is a sticky and colorless film of bacteria and sugars that constantly forms on our teeth. The bacteria use ingredients found in our diet and saliva to grow. The film starts forming just 1 or 2 minutes after brushing your teeth. This is why we need to brush at least twice a day to continue removing these bacteria.

Think of plaque like peanut butter on a knife. Plopping a knife smeared with peanut butter in some water probably isn't going to clean it very well. Peanut butter is too sticky. Plaque acts like peanut butter on your teeth. The major difference between the two is that the peanut butter isn't damaging that knife. The plaque, however, is doing serious damage to your teeth. Plaque starts to harden in just 48 hours and begins turning into tartar (or dental calculus, as dentists call it). After approximately ten days, that tartar is rock hard and difficult to remove, collecting at the gum line. Then brushing and flossing become more difficult. As the tartar, plaque, and bacteria continue to increase, cavities can form, and gums become inflamed. This inflammation causes gums to become red and swollen, and they may begin to bleed.

How do I know if my child's teeth are clean?

Although plaque is colorless and difficult to see at first, when plaque builds up, it looks like a thick white film stuck to the teeth. You can also feel plaque on your teeth with your tongue. The plaque biofilm feels like a sticky layer of fuzz or fur. Clean teeth should feel slick and smooth as you run your tongue across them.

If you want to know if your child's tooth-brushing regimen is effective, buy a plaque-disclosing tablet. They are relatively inexpensive and be found at your local pharmacy or online. The tablets are usual of vegetable dye and are very easy to use. Once the tablet dis mouth, it temporarily stains the plaque bright red, blue, you can see it more easily. You can then brush and f gone. Your child will remember what the color will know where to brush better from then o

How to Brush Your Child's T

You will need to help with old, to be sure all surfaces a gums, and mouth in little ci bing horizontally can create groo

Also be careful not to brush too hard. Many people think that the harder they brush, the cleaner they can get their teeth, but this is not true. Hard brushing can damage tooth surfaces.

1. Wash your hands first, to make sure you get rid of any germs you may be carrying around. It is often easiest to cradle your child's head in your one arm while keeping your other hand free to brush. Brush the teeth from behind, which will help you reach the top and bottom rows. Place the toothbrush alongside the teeth, with the bristles at a 45-degree angle to the gum line.

2. Gently move the brush in a small circular motion, cleaning the front surface of one tooth at time. Be sure to follow a system so you don't miss any teeth. You can start with the bottom back tooth and work your way to the front, then repeat on the opposite side of the mouth before switching to the top teeth.

3. Brush across the chewing surfaces, making sure the bristles get into the grooves and crevices. Clean the side of the teeth that face the tongue using the same circular motion. Again, start in the back and work your way forward. Move the "toe" of the brush up and down to clean inside front teeth.

Brush your child's tongue lightly ove bacteria and keep breath good.

your child rinse her mouth

her every time you her teeth by clapping ing.

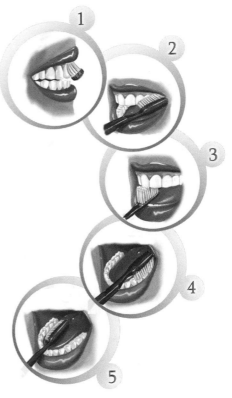

This is the correct method and toothbrush angle to use when brushing teeth. Make sure to reach every tooth surface. Courtesy of Alila Sao Mai / Shutterstock.com

*Cleaning my daughter's tongue seems a little gross.
Is it really necessary?*

Although you can buy a tongue scraper to remove bacteria and food particles clinging to your child's tongue, a special tool isn't necessary. A quick couple of swipes with the toothbrush are just as effective to remove bacteria, alleviate bad breath, and cut down on cavities and gum disease. It takes just an extra few seconds for an added boost of oral health.

How long should tooth brushing take?

Each day, on average people spend 8.5 hours sleeping, 1 hour eating, 7.2 minutes volunteering, and only 50 seconds brushing their teeth. Dentists recommend brushing for at least 2 or 3 minutes each time we brush. Without making any changes in your child's normal routine, grab a timer and secretly record just how long your child's average tooth brushing lasts. You might be surprised.

Want to boost the brushing? Let her favorite pop star's newest release be the tooth-brushing anthem. Most songs are 2 or 3 minutes long. When it starts, so does the brushing. She can't stop until the song is done. For younger children, get a timer or a musical toothbrush that lets you know when the time is up.

Two Minutes, Two Times

For more ideas about how to get your kids to brush for at least two minutes two times at day, visit www.2min2x.org This interactive Web site, sponsored by the Partnership for Healthy Mouths, Healthy Lives, contains lots of games, videos, rewards, and other fun materials to get children excited about keeping their teeth clean.

Can You Brush Too Much?

Yes, you can brush your child's teeth too heavily, too much, or in the wrong way. Rubbing the toothbrush as hard as you can against the teeth or gums can be damaging. It can destroy tooth enamel, making teeth look yellow, or push up the gums, causing them to weaken and recede. Learning good brushing habits and techniques is important for protecting your child's teeth. If you are unsure, your dentist or dental hygienist will be happy to show you.

How often should I brush my child's teeth?

Most dentists suggest brushing at least twice a day. Ideally, we would all brush after every snack and meal. Try to get your child in the habit of at

least rinsing with water within 10 minutes of eating or drinking, to help minimize acid destruction
to teeth and gums. Although brushing is always
best, rinsing with water can be helpful in a pinch.
It will not remove plaque, but it should help get rid
of debris on the teeth.

Keep a bag with a tube of toothpaste and disposable toothbrushes (or a toothbrush with a cap)
in your car and in your child's school backpack to
make it easier to brush on the go. Although your
child may not use it often, seeing the toothbrush is
a good reminder to make tooth-friendly choices.

> *Set a Good Example*
>
> Make sure your child sees you brushing your teeth throughout the day, and make a point of show-ing off your shiny, clean teeth. Ham it up with your best grin to show what a treat and privilege it is to have such a shiny smile. Encourage your child to show off his own sparkly smile after brushing.

At the very least, your child's teeth should be brushed in the morning and
before bedtime and after eating sweet or sticky foods. Any other times are
healthy bonuses.

How do I teach my child to brush her own teeth?

As your child grows, always talk about what you're doing when you
brush her teeth. Teach her to put the brush at a 45-degree angle against her
gums; move it back and forth gently in wide strokes over all teeth; move the
"toe" of the brush up and down to clean inside front teeth; and brush her
tongue gently to remove bacteria and freshen breath. In no time, she'll be
able to carry on the family tradition of cleaning her teeth well.

When should I let my son brush his own teeth?

You can begin to teach your child proper brushing techniques when
he is about 2 or 3 years old. Follow up with brushing and gentle flossing
until age 7 or 8, when he has the dexterity to do it alone. Allow younger
children to brush first, then follow up with your more thorough cleaning
until you are sure they can do it alone. Most children cannot floss well on
their own until they reach age 9 or 10.

How to Find and Care for Toothbrushes

What kind of toothbrush should I choose for my child?

From glow-in-the-dark to singing, there are dozens of different types of toothbrushes on the market for children. The average toothbrush is plastic and has around 2,500 bristles grouped into about 40 tufts. Whether they are motorized or not or have tons of special features, most toothbrushes do a pretty good job of removing plaque. Check the label for the ADA seal as well as for the recommended age to ensure the appropriate size and bristle softness for your child. Choose a toothbrush with

- a small brush head that will fit in your child's mouth
- an angled head to clean hard-to-reach places
- a flexible neck to absorb brushing pressure that may cause gum irritation
- a large handle for a secure grip whether it is wet or dry

There are electric toothbrushes with vibrating heads available for children to help remove plaque and debris. Some dentists believe that these toothbrushes are more effective in removing plaque, but there's little data to support this. The best toothbrush for children is one that they like and will use often.

Keep in mind your child's preferences and particular needs. For example, a child with sensory issues might love (or hate) an electric toothbrush, while a child with small hands or poor fine motor skills might do better with a large, easy-to-grip, or flexible handle. If it's in your budget, specialty toothbrushes decorated with favorite characters, colors, or sparkles may generate more toothbrushing enthusiasm, at least in the short term.

What Is the ADA Seal?

When browsing the toothbrush aisle, look for the ADA seal on toothbrushes, which means they have met the minimum standards set by the American Dental Association. The ADA does not recommend any specific brand of toothbrush, but it does give its seal of approval to brands that meet basic standards. The ADA seal indicates that the toothbrush is effective for cleaning teeth and safe for a child to use without adult supervision—the bristles have no sharp or jagged edges or endpoints, the handle won't break during normal use, and the bristles won't fall out. The seal also indicates that the brush has been evaluated by scientists to show that it provides a "significant decrease in mild periodontal disease and plaque."

I just leave all the toothbrushes in a jar on the bathroom counter.
Is that ok?

Simply allow your toothbrush to air-dry and then store it in an upright position. Do not cover your toothbrush, such as with a cap, because humid air is more likely to promote bacterial growth. Storing toothbrushes some space apart from each other will reduce the possibility of cross-contamination, especially important for people with compromised immune systems or infectious diseases. If multiple brushes are stored in the same holder, do not allow them to come in contact with each other. It may sound obvious, but keep your toothbrush container away from the toilet. If someone flushes the toilet with the lid up, the particulate can spray and reach those brushes. Keep those brushes far away from the flushes!

Everyone should have his or her own toothbrush, and if your kids' brushes look alike, clearly label each brush with the name of its owner. Do not allow toothbrush sharing, because it puts everyone at an increased risk for cross-contamination. Family members can become infected with all kinds of bacteria if they share toothbrushes.

> ### Nontoxic Toothbrushes
>
> Many parents want to avoid any products that contain bisphenol-A (BPA), PVC, or phthalates due to increasing concerns about the potential harmful effects of these chemicals on growing bodies. If you want your little ones brushing in nontoxic style, look for toothbrushes made from polypropylene (#5) and nylon (for the bristles).

A friend of mine soaks her family's toothbrushes in mouthwash
every week. Should I do that?

Toothbrush care is pretty simple, and you don't need to soak your toothbrushes in mouthwash. It won't hurt your toothbrush if you do, but soaking your whole family's brushes in the same bowl of mouthwash can spread the bacteria from brush to brush.

Rinsing the brush with warm water after brushing is surprisingly effective. Bleaching a toothbrush leaves a chlorine residue on the bristles that can affect the taste the next time the brush is used. Soaking a toothbrush in hot water from the faucet or in the dishwasher will cause the bristles to degrade and reduce the life of the brush.

Researchers have found that microwaving toothbrushes kills common germs; however, the metal staples that hold the bristles in the manual toothbrush head can interfere with the energy waves and destroy the microwave. Experts caution that microwave sterilization is not a good idea. After all, new toothbrushes cost a lot less than new microwaves.

You can buy a toothbrush sanitizer, although be aware that some manufacturers make claims not yet widely accepted. The U.S. Food and Drug Administration (FDA) allows manufacturers to make only these two claims for toothbrush sanitizers: (1) the product is designed to sanitize toothbrushes, and (2) the product is intended for use in reducing bacterial contamination that accumulates naturally on toothbrushes. Claims that go beyond these are largely unsubstantiated. A good rinse in warm water after brushing should serve your purposes equally well.

How often should I replace toothbrushes?

Remember—this piece of plastic is the foundation of your family's oral care. This is not the place to skimp. Plan to replace everyone's toothbrush every three to four months, or when the toothbrush bristles become splayed or spread out. According to the American Dental Association, replacing your brush this often is based on the expected wear of the toothbrush, not on its bacterial contamination. A worn toothbrush is less effective in doing its job—cleaning teeth and removing plaque.

Note that toothbrushes are not required to be sold in sterile packages, so rinse your toothbrush in warm water before using it the first time. Also, replace your toothbrush (or your child's) any time

Recycle Your Toothbrush

What can you do with an old toothbrush? We all go through several per year. You could pull out the bristles, boil it for an hour, and mold it into a bracelet or use it for other craft projects. For the less creative, old toothbrushes make great cleaning tools for hard-to-reach places (just soak it in disinfectant first). Some toothbrushes now have handles made from recyclable plastics. These can be put in your recycle bin at home and will then be melted down and repurposed. Next time you buy a toothbrush, look for the recycle symbol on the packaging.

after having a sore throat or other illness so that you do not risk reinfecting yourself or infecting your children.

How to Find the Right Toothpaste

Are all toothpastes the same?

There are almost as many kinds of toothpaste on the market as there are types of toothbrushes, but choosing the right toothpaste for your child isn't as complicated as it looks.

Most of the toothpastes designed for specific purposes like gingivitis control, tartar control, and whitening are made for adults and aren't ideal for children. Some parents look for the American Dental Association (ADA) seal, which shows that the association has tested the product and says that it is safe and effective.

Regardless of what kind of toothpaste you choose, make sure your child does not swallow it. Help him develop the habit of spitting out the paste, to reduce the risk of developing white spots on the teeth (called fluorosis) or swallowing too much of the fluoride contained in toothpaste, because too much fluoride can also be harmful.

Some children need prescription toothpaste to help protect against cavities. (Health insurance *may* help cover the cost.) Prescription-strength fluoride toothpaste contains a higher concentration of fluoride than regular toothpaste. It may be prescribed to children who frequently develop cavities, who get little fluoride, or who are at higher risk for tooth decay. Read the directions carefully. Some dentists suggest that the prescription toothpaste be used only once a day,

> *What's in Toothpaste?*
>
> Toothpaste is made up of about 20 to 42 percent water. The other main components include abrasives, which account for about 50 percent of the toothpaste and are insoluble particles that help remove plaque from the teeth; fluoride, which helps to prevent cavities; and detergents, which mainly serve as foaming agents and enable the uniform distribution of toothpaste, improving its cleansing power. Additional components may include antibacterial agents to prevent gingivitis and reduce tartar and bad breath; flavorants, which improve the taste and therefore encourage brushing; remineralizers to help re-form the enamel; and other miscellaneous components that are usually added to prevent the toothpaste from drying out, reduce sensitivity, whiten teeth, or further minimize the formation of tartar.

> *How Much Toothpaste?*
>
> For young children, a pea-sized squirt is all you need.

and then regular toothpaste for the rest of the day's brushings. Note that the ADA does not offer a seal program for prescription toothpaste products.

Is it harmful to swallow toothpaste?

It is important for children to learn the skill of spitting out toothpaste. Until they can do so, make sure you use a nonfluoridated or low-fluoridated toothpaste. Most toothpaste contains about 1,000 to 1,500 parts per million fluoride. Children under 6 should be offered toothpaste with fluoride in the lower ranges, in case they inadvertently swallow a large amount. Fluoride is fine for your child in moderation, but fluoridated toothpaste should not be regularly swallowed.

Too much fluoride can cause fluorosis, marked by discolored spots on the teeth. Talk to your dentist about the amount of fluoride in your water,

> *Hold a*
> *Toothpaste Taste Test*
>
> Want to generate some enthusiasm for tooth brushing? Buy several different brands and flavors of toothpaste and hold a taste test. Try a new one every night or have a tooth-brushing frenzy and try them all in an evening.

Fluoride: What Parents Need to Know

Fluoride is a mineral that prevents tooth decay and helps harden tooth enamel. Because very few foods contain fluoride, most people get the mineral through fluoridated water, toothpastes, and sometimes even supplements when needed. Fluoride is important for oral health, and inadequate amounts can significantly increase the risk for tooth decay. However, fluoride can be toxic if consumed in excessive amounts. This often causes parents to wonder if fluoride is even safe, especially since some critics have linked it to cancer.

The Centers for Disease Control and Prevention and the American Dental Association concluded in 2001 that "when used appropriately, fluoride is a safe and effective agent that can be used to prevent and control tooth decay. Fluoride has contributed profoundly to the improved dental health of persons in the United States and other countries. To ensure additional improvements in oral health among all children, water fluoridation should be extended to additional communities, and fluoride toothpaste should be used widely." Furthermore, the American Cancer Society asserts that there is no strong evidence for a link between cancer and fluoride.

To protect your child's teeth, talk with his dentist about how much fluoride your child is getting based on environment, diet, and other factors. (For more information about fluoride, see chapter 4, Preventing Decay and Protecting Teeth.)

Sensitivity Alert

Some people are sensitive to the foaming agent found in some toothpastes, and they develop mouth sores. If your child tries a new toothpaste and develops a tender spot on the inside of his mouth, it might be sodium laureth (or lauryl) sulfate, or SLS, that's to blame. Commercial toothpastes usually contain SLS, but you can find SLS-free options at most health food stores. If not, a quick online search will yield several options.

and ask if your child should avoid fluoride-added toothpaste. If so, it's easy to find toothpastes that do not contain fluoride by reading toothpaste labels carefully. You may have to go to a natural foods store or order toothpaste online.

Are there gluten-free toothpastes?

Many toothpastes are gluten-free, although not all companies are willing to certify that their products are gluten-free because they may be manufactured in facilities the make products containing gluten. You may need to pay extra for certified gluten-free products. Contact your child's dentist before your visit to let the staff know about your child's gluten sensitivity. Most products used in dental offices are gluten-free, but the dental staff should be made aware of your child's needs.

Seven manufacturers verify that all their toothpastes are gluten-free.

- Aquafresh
- Arm & Hammer
- Crest
- Nature's Gate
- Orajel
- Oral-B
- Tom's of Maine

What if my child hates the taste of toothpaste?

Is Baking Soda Dangerous to Enamel?

Some people worry that, because baking soda is so effective as a cleaning polish, it may take the enamel off teeth along with plaque. But it's brushing too vigorously, particularly brushing horizontally, that's hard on the teeth and gums. So whether you're brushing with baking soda or regular toothpaste, the important thing is to brush in little circles and not horizontally.

Toothpaste should be at least pleasant for children. Some people have more sensitive palates than others, and flavors that are okay for some are disgusting to others. For years, bubble gum was the only available kid's flavor, but the choices are expanding. Look to online drugstores for a host of flavors, including light salt, tropical, peppermint, fresh yogurt, rose, monkey banana, honey, cafe au lait, apple, vanilla, strawberry, orange, green tea, lavender, cinnamon, lemon tea, bitter chocolate, blueberry, caramel, espresso, grapefruit, and cola. Even the pickiest child can find an appealing flavor on that list. Flavored toothpaste won't hurt as long as your child doesn't eat it.

Another option is to make your own toothpaste. You might find that your child pays more attention to dental care and brushing because you've worked together to make the toothpaste. Making your own toothpaste can be messy, however, and many people agree that it doesn't always taste that great either.

> ### What's in Homemade Toothpaste?
>
> *Ingredients*
> 4 teaspoons baking soda
> 1 teaspoon sea or kosher salt
> 1 teaspoon flavoring (vanilla, almond, or peppermint extract)
> Xylitol (optional)
> Air-tight container
>
> *Directions*
> Mix the ingredients together and use as needed. Be sure to cover the container with a tight-fitting lid after each use. To limit exposure to bacteria, make sure you use a container that won't require you to dip your toothbrush into it every time you want to use it.

Is toothpaste even necessary?

As we said before, dental plaque is like peanut butter smeared on your teeth. Water alone won't get it off. The most effective way to remove that sticky plaque is to scrape it off with a good soft-bristled brush, water, and lots of gentle scrubbing action, followed by flossing. Toothpaste isn't

> ### The History of Toothpaste
>
> In 5000 BC, Egyptians were making a tooth powder consisting of myrrh, pumice, and even powdered ashes of ox hooves or powdered and burnt eggshells. Using their fingers, they rubbed the powder on their teeth. The Greeks improved the recipes by adding abrasives like crushed bones and oyster shells, which helped remove debris from teeth. Later, the Romans, concerned about bad breath, added powdered charcoal, powdered bark, and more flavoring agents. In 1000 AD, the Persians advised their people to be wary of the possible dangers of using hard abrasives as tooth powders. It was recommended that people use burnt hartshorn, the burnt shells of snails, and burnt gypsum. Other Persian recipes involved dried animal parts, herbs, honey, and minerals.

Dry Brush Your Teeth

If you want to be extra thorough, dry brush your teeth without toothpaste first. Do it before you brush with toothpaste and water and you'll cut tartar by 60 percent and reduce the risk of bleeding gums by about 50 percent. Use a dry, soft brush to scrub the insides of your top and bottom teeth, then buff the outer and front surfaces. Rinse, spit, and then brush again with toothpaste.

absolutely necessary, but it is helpful. It tastes good and makes your mouth feel fresh and clean. And for most children, the added fluoride in toothpaste helps keep tooth enamel hard and cavity resistant. So you don't need it, but toothpaste is a good investment for a healthy smile. Whatever kind you use, limit the amount to pea-sized.

Should I use natural products?

Toothpaste is an artificial product, created with different blends of chemicals, additives, and flavorings. Some parents may wish to avoid certain chemicals in their children's diets, even though children ingest a relatively small amount of product. You can easily find toothpastes for children that contain no saccharin or other artificial sweeteners, preservatives, colors, or flavors, or animal ingredients. You can even find certified kosher or vegan toothpaste.

There are "natural" toothbrushes on the market as well. Most toothbrush bristles are made from nylon, but some companies have created bristles made from the root of trees and other products. You might find toothbrushes with brown bristles that are reportedly softer than nylon bristles. Although such toothbrushes won't hurt your teeth, there's no indication that forking over more money will translate into better oral care.

Flossing and Mouthwash

Do I really need to floss my child's teeth?

Few people love flossing. Most Americans admit they would rather grocery shop than floss their teeth. But it's an important part of your child's (and your) dental routine. Even the best tooth brushing touches only 70 percent of tooth surfaces. Flossing

Floss is Handy to Have Around

Keep lots of dental floss at your house. In a pinch, dental floss works well as a cake cutter, makeshift clothesline, fishing line, picture hanger, and more. If flossing properly, the average person should use 122 yards of floss per year. About a third of adults claim to floss daily, but sales data show an average of only 18 yards of floss are sold per person a year, so our dental habits aren't as good as we report.

removes plaque and food particles caught between teeth, where multiple cavities can form if you are just brushing alone.

Your child should be able to floss her own teeth by about 8 or 9 years old. Until then, flossing is a parent's job. You should start flossing your child's teeth as soon as she has two teeth that touch each other.

What kind of dental floss is best for kids?

Dental floss comes in many different forms, including a flosser (a short piece of floss held by a small plastic "y"), an electric flosser, unwaxed or waxed floss, and woven and shred-resistant floss. There are even brightly colored kid-friendly flossers decorated with the likes of princesses, sea creatures, and super heroes. Like toothbrushes and toothpaste, the kind your child will use most is the best kind for him. Flossers can be tricky to use in the back of the mouth once molars arrive, and you'll have to wipe off the plaque after each use. Waxed flosses or dental "gloss" are often easiest to work in between tight teeth, but otherwise, most dental flosses are fine for children.

Flossing Correctly

1. Take about 18 inches of dental floss and wrap one end around each of your middle fingers.

2. Using your thumbs and index fingers as guides, slide the floss between two teeth, using a gentle saw-like motion.

3. At the gum line, pull both ends of the floss in the same direction to form a C shape against one tooth. Pull the floss tightly and move it up and down against one tooth.

4. Pull the floss against the other tooth and repeat the motion.

5. Repeat this for all teeth. Be sure to floss both sides of the teeth farthest back in the mouth, too.

Is Cupcake-Covered Dental Floss a Bad Idea?

You can choose from dozens of dental floss flavors, though you have to find the more esoteric ones online. Who wouldn't want to floss with the flavor of crispy fried bacon or vanilla cupcakes? Flavored dental floss seems like a great idea. After all, who can argue about a product that makes children want to floss their teeth? Keep in mind, though, that some children will like the flavor so much they'll want to chew on it, and it's easy to swallow if a caregiver isn't supervising closely. Although it's likely that what goes in will eventually come out the other end, more than one child has had to have an endoscopy to remove a mass of tangled floss

Should my child use mouthwash?

Mouthwashes are not necessary for young children. In fact, sometimes people who use mouthwash do a less thorough job of tooth brushing, assuming that mouthwash covers a multitude of sins. It can taste good and can help give a just-brushed feeling, but it doesn't help remove plaque.

If you decide to buy mouthwash for your child, look for one designed for children, because it is more likely to have a pleasing flavor and it won't contain alcohol, as many adult versions do. Some dentists may recommend an antibacterial mouthwash for short-term use in children who are especially susceptible to cavities. Regardless of the kind, always supervise when your child uses mouthwash. Children under age 6 should not use mouthwash at all because they have a harder time swishing and spitting and are more likely to swallow it.

> ### *Lock Up Your Mouthwash*
> If you buy mouthwash designed for adults, look for alcohol-free versions, and choose bottles with child-proof caps. Children have had to be rushed to the hospital after ingesting alcohol-laden mouthwash. After all, it's brightly colored, easily accessible, and designed to taste good. Always keep it in a safe place, away from curious little ones.

CHAPTER 3

The Dental Visit

Like most parents, Leslie had a running internal list of things she need-ed to do. Between writing a check for piano lessons and signing the field trip permission slip, she remembered the crumpled reminder notice from the dentist. Both kids were now way overdue for their six-month checkup. She sighed, mentally pushing aside the note and promising herself that she'd deal with it tomorrow.

Admittedly, it's hard to be enthusiastic about going to the dentist. With the inconvenience, expense, previous personal experiences, and our often unfounded fears about our children's discomfort, we can easily talk our-selves into postponing regular dental visits for our kids. But considering how important oral care is to your child's overall health, those regular den-tist visits are every bit as important as regular pediatrician visits, where your child gets immunizations and checkups. Routine dental checkups are the cornerstone of your child's oral health.

How to Find a Dentist

Picking the first dentist that a Google search turns up isn't the best plan. Although that dentist may be excellent, he or she may also have been the only one in your area to pay Google for advertising. A willingness to spend money on ads says nothing about quality, no matter how nice the ads are. Consider several factors when looking for a new dentist for your child. Start with making a list of your specific preferences and needs. These questions might help you figure those out.

- What does the "right" dentist mean to you? Does it mean an office that's convenient to your work or your child's school? One that's open on Saturday or late in the day to fit your schedule? One that reminds you of your dentist growing up, or where you get a live person whenever you call instead of an answering service?
- Is the dentist up to date on the latest in cutting-edge pediatric dental treatments?
- Is your child more comfortable around certain types of people, such as men or women or those that are more quiet and gentle or more talkative and animated?
- Does your child have fears about the dentist or other special needs?

After you have made a list of what's important to you, it's easier to match your needs with the right dentist for your child. Here are some other factors to consider.

Referrals. Ask around. Who does your pediatrician recommend? Who does your neighbor recommend? How about other parents in the Scout troop? Are there dentists they recommend and dentists they don't recommend? Ask about their experiences and what they did and didn't like about the dental practice. You're looking for more than a dentist—you need to know about the office staff and dental hygienists, too. You can contact the local or state dental society or a local community listing. If you're moving, your current dentist may be able to make a recommendation for a dentist in your new area.

Insurance. Is this dentist in or out of your dental insurance network? Can office staff assist patients in working with their insurance companies? Will they precertify with the insurance company for procedures, or will you need to do that? Will they bill your insurance, or will you have to pay at the time of the visit and then get reimbursed?

Policies. You want to know what the policies are for emergencies *before* you're holding a broken tooth in the middle of a soccer field on a Saturday afternoon. Do they have emergency hours or an emergency contact number? What is their cancellation policy? Children are unpredictable. If your child wakes up with the flu on the morning of a dental appointment, you don't want to be surprised with a $50 cancellation fee.

Should I call a dental referral company?

Use a referral company with care. Dental referral companies prescreen participants, and they generally can supply you with information on the dentists' educational background, experience, and specialty. They can usually provide other information as well, such as a dentist who can speak a second language or who has the specific office hours you want. Be aware, however, that most of these services list only dentists who pay to be included.

> *The Pediatric Dentist Locator Service*
>
> The American Academy of Pediatric Dentistry's (AAPD) online Find a Pediatric Dentist service provides quick access to information on pediatric dentists for the general public. The directory is updated weekly and contains the names, addresses, telephone numbers, and fax numbers of pediatric dentists in the United States who are members in good standing of the AAPD. Simply type in your zip code and the search radius (from 5 to 150 miles) in the Find a Pediatric Dentist search box at www.aapd.org.

What questions should I ask dentists to help me choose the right one?

After you've come up with a list of two or three dentists, consider whether they are conveniently located. If their offices are not near where you live or work, you may have trouble keeping appointments. Next, call their offices and ask some preliminary questions:

- At what age does the dentist recommend seeing patients for their first visit?
- Does the dentist regularly treat children or patients with special health care needs?
- Is the office child-friendly, including the waiting room and the treatment areas?
- What are the office hours? (Is the dentist available when you're available?)
- Does the practice accept your dental plan?

- Is payment requested at each visit, or will the dentist file a claim with your insurance company and bill you for the balance?
  - What are the fees for standard treatments (e.g., x-rays or cleaning)?
  - Is information about fees provided before treatment is scheduled, including a pretreatment estimate?
  - Is the practice willing to set up a payment plan for more expensive treatments? Will they work with you to come up with a plan you can afford?
  - Does the dental staff use universal precautions for infection control, such as gloves, masks, protective clothing, and sterilized instruments and work areas?
  - What is the protocol for patients who have emergencies during office hours, after office hours, or when the dentist is away?
  - If you call the practice with a problem, can you speak to the dentist? Are there established times for calls to and from the dentist? Are telephone calls returned the same day?
  - Are patients notified when it's time for a checkup? Will you receive a reminder call, text, or e-mail the day before a scheduled appointment? (This can be a very helpful service.)
  - Does the dental office have a Web site? How much information is shared online or through e-mail?

If you like what you hear, schedule an appointment for a meet-and-greet with the dentist. Taking the time to meet a dentist can help you gauge if the person and office is a good fit for your family. If possible, bring your child to meet the new dentist.

Be sure to ask plenty of questions. For example, if your child is anxious about dental visits, ask what techniques are available to soothe children. Ask about dental emergency hours. And while you're there, take a good look around. Look for special amenities like toys, designated play areas, and TVs in the treatment rooms. Special touches can help calm even the most anxious child and can give you insight into the office's attitude toward

---

DDS or DMD?

Some dentists have DDS after their names, while others have DMD. DDS stands for doctor of dental surgery, and DMD stands for doctor of dental medicine. Because of standardized regulation of U.S. dental schools, there is no difference in the educational qualifications of a dentist with a DDS degree and one with a DMD degree. Today, the degrees simply indicate the history of the dental school.

accommodating the needs of children. If you cannot tour the office in advance, then see if you can view the office on the dentist's Web site. Many dental practices include photographs of the office and their staff online.

Types of Dentists

What is a pediatric dentist?

A pediatric dentist is a specialized type of dentist just for infants, children, and teens, like a pediatrician for teeth. In addition to a four-year college education, then dental school, pediatric dentists complete two to three years of additional specialized training focused on dentistry for children. This focus includes extra attention to proper care of baby teeth and permanent teeth, once they start to erupt. Although general dentists are certainly capable of treating children, pediatric dentists have chosen this field because they are passionate about working with little ones. Pediatric dentistry is one of the fastest growing specialties for dentists.

> **A Growing Field**
> Pediatric dentistry is the fastest growing dental specialty in the United States.

Besides their additional training, pediatric dentists often have dental offices designed with children's comfort in mind. From books, toys, and DVD players to pillows, blankets, and themed treatment rooms, every effort is made to help your little ones feel safe and cared for.

What other dental specialties are there?

Understanding dental specialties can be confusing. Family, or general, dentists can be an appropriate choice for children's oral care needs. These dentists focus on the diagnosis and treatment of dental problems in people at any age. There are several advantages to using a family dentist, including having the entire family cared for by one office, a convenient location, and, in some cases, lower fees. Some general dentists have received additional training in working with children and consider them a valuable part of their practice, while others prefer to focus on adults.

Orthodontics is a branch of dentistry many families with children encounter. Orthodontists specialize in preventing and treating tooth and facial irregularities, including problems with bites, jaw alignment, tooth crowding, and more. Treatment involves braces, retainers, and other cor-rective "appliances." Some pediatric dentists have additional training in orthodontics, providing a "one-stop shop" for patients, while others refer patients to a specialist for orthodontic work.

Endodontics is a dental specialty that deals with diseases inside the tooth that affect tissue, blood vessels, and nerves. The most common endodontic treatment is a root canal—the removal of infected tissue and refilling of the nerve canal inside the tooth.

Oral surgery is the specialty involving surgical treatment of diseases, injuries, and deformities of the mouth, teeth, gums, and jaws. This in-cludes treating problems caused by wisdom teeth, facial injuries, and jaw disorders. Oral surgeons are also skilled in re-constructive and dental implant surgery.

Periodontics refers to the diagnosis and treat-ment, including gum surgery, of problems with the gums and bone that hold teeth in place.

Prosthodontics, also called prosthetic dentistry, involves replacing teeth with artificial substitutes, or false teeth. Prosthodontists often work with tooth replacement implants, crowns and bridges, partial dentures, and complete dentures.

Cosmetic dentistry is another term used by dentists which generally refers to any dental work that improves the appearance (although not nec-essarily the function) of a person's teeth or bite.

> **Green Dentists**
>
> Some dentists have made a concerted effort to decrease the environmental effects of their dental practices by using digital x-rays, elec-tronic charting, and eco-friendly products. If you are interested in finding a dentist committed to incor-porating green practices in the office, look for a certi-fied green dentist at the Eco-Dentistry Association, www.ecodentistry.org.

What do dental hygienists and dental assistants do?

Dental hygienists are licensed health care providers who specialize in preventing and treating oral diseases. Before they can practice, they must graduate from an accredited dental hygiene program and pass written and clinical exams. Dental hygienists play a key role in the oral health care of their clients through in-office preventive services and education about home care. They are great resources for oral health care tips—from more effective brushing and flossing techniques to selecting oral health care products.

Your dental office may also employ dental assistants. They usually assist the dentist or dental hygienist in preparing the patient for treatment, sterilizing instruments, passing instruments to the dentist during the procedure, holding a suction device, doing dental x-rays, taking impressions, and getting crowns ready. Their help enables dentists and dental hygienists to focus more time on the procedure and provide more efficient dental treatments. Dental assistants are regulated on a state-by-state basis, so there could be differences in how dental assistants are trained or what they can do depending on your state.

Private Dental Hygienists

In rural and underserved areas across the country, dental hygienists have gone into private practice to offer cleanings for less cost than a typical dentist visit. Although the fees are much less, they do not include x-rays or other screenings— only a cleaning is provided. If you want more frequent cleanings, these offices may offer a helpful service, but keep in mind that these cleanings should be done in addition to, and not replace, regular dental exams.

Preparing for Your Child's First Visit

Why does our dentist need to know our family's health history and my child's medical history?

Most dentists ask you to fill out a medical history form on your first visit to their office. All of this information helps decrease the likelihood of complications during dental treatments. Take the time to read over each question and answer it accurately. You should always inform the dentist of all existing medical conditions, treatments, and medications. Let your child's dentist know about diabetes, allergies, and medications for kidney, lung, heart, or liver disease. Also, be honest about your child's habits, such as eating choices and smoking, including exposure to secondhand smoke. Update your child's records at each visit if there are any changes to health status or medications.

Certain medications or conditions may affect the way your child's teeth react to treatment. For example, pregnancy may increase the risk of gum disease, and bleeding gums and arthritis can make it difficult for patients to maintain a clean mouth. If your child's dentist and staff don't know about underlying problems, they run the risk of performing unsuccessful treatments.

Expect to answer these questions, or similar ones, regarding your child's health history:

- What was the date and purpose of your child's last visit to a doctor?
- Does your child suffer from any disability? If yes, describe.
- Has your child ever taken or been exposed to illegal drugs? If yes, what drugs and when taken?
- Is your child HIV-positive or does your child have hepatitis?
- List all medications your child is now taking or has taken previously on a regular basis; describe the strength and purpose for each.
- Has your child ever had an allergic reaction to medication? If yes, describe.
- Describe any surgeries your child has had.
- Is your child on a special diet? If yes, for what reason? Describe the diet.
- Does your child smoke? If yes, describe type and quantity.
- Has your child consulted or been treated by a psychiatrist, psychologist, or counselor? If yes, when and for what purpose?
- Are you aware of any other concerns about your child's health?
- For children under 10 years old: Was your child born by Cesarean section? Was your child born full term or premature?
- Is your child allergic to latex? If yes, what was the reaction?
- Has your child ever been treated for (or with):
  - Rheumatic fever, rheumatic heart disease, heart murmur, or congenital heart disease?
  - Heart trouble, heart attack, angina, heart surgery, a pacemaker, or irregular beats?
  - Stomach or intestinal disease?
  - Breathing problems, asthma, tuberculosis, or hay fever?
  - Diabetes?
  - Kidney problems or renal dialysis?
  - Tumors or growths?
  - Arthritis or rheumatism?

∘ Behavioral problems such as ADHD (attention deficit hyperactivity disorder), ODD (oppositional defiant disorder), PDD (pervasive developmental disorder), or autism spectrum disorder?

If you are concerned about how the information will be used or who will have access to the information, speak to the dentist or the office manager directly. Dentists are required to protect all health information in the same way that other health care providers do because of the strict HIPAA privacy rule, which protects the privacy of individually identifiable health information. You have the right to feel confident that the information you share will be protected.

What is included in an initial dental cleaning or basic checkup?

Checkups usually include a complete cleaning, by either the dentist or a dental hygienist. Using special instruments, the dentist or hygienist will gently scrape below the gum line, removing built-up plaque and tartar that can cause gum disease, cavities, bad breath, and other problems. Your child's dentist or hygienist may also polish and floss your child's teeth and possibly apply a fluoride solution.

After reviewing your child's medical and dental history, the dentist will perform a thorough examination of your child's teeth, gums, and mouth, looking for signs of disease or other problems. The goal is to help maintain your child's good oral health and to prevent problems from becoming serious by identifying and treating them as soon as possible.

The dentist will first look in your child's mouth using a mirror and perhaps a light, looking for staining, cracked or broken teeth, and cavities as well as counting how many teeth there are. The dentist or an assisting staff member will chart the findings, using the number or letter assigned to each tooth. Then the dentist will use a dental probe, called an explorer, to gently feel the bumps and valleys on the surface of each tooth. Any tackiness or stickiness on the surface might be a soft area indicating decay. Some dentists have a device called diagnodent, a gentle light device that rests on the tooth and shines a light that reveals any decay. Teeth usually need to be cleaned first, to remove debris and allow the device to work properly. Some dentists use an intra-oral camera, a form of video examination, which allows both the doctor and the patient (and the patient's caregiver) to see the condition of the mouth at the same time, and then discuss treatment options.

How do I prepare my child for a first dental visit?

It may help to explain to your child that the dentist is a friendly person who helps take care of children's teeth. After all, going to the dentist is an exciting part of growing up. Emphasize the positive parts of the visit. You could explain to your child that the dentist will count his teeth, clean them with a special tickling toothbrush, and take some pictures of his mouth. Never tell your child that the dentist will not "hurt" him, for that may have never even occurred to him. Don't bribe your child into going to the dentist—this only makes it seem like there must be danger ahead. Visit the American Dental Association Web site (www.ada.org) with your child for games and stories to prepare him for his dental visit.

Should I go back with my child or let her go alone?

Some dental offices prefer that children go alone once they are school age. Most pediatric dentists, however, encourage parents to sit with their children during appointments. If you choose to accompany your child, most dental offices suggest that you be a silent observer. Offer a hand to hold if needed, but let the staff be the ones who direct your child's movements. It is important for the dentist and staff to establish cooperation and trust directly with your child, and your child may become easily confused if more than one person is speaking to her. Look for a dental practice that considers it important to gain children's friendship and trust and where they use all their resources to achieve this goal.

Ideally, a dental practice will implement the Tell, Show, Do method, where staff members explain everything to your child in age-appropriate terms, demonstrate what they are going to do, then do it. If you are with your child, follow the dentist's instructions closely. If you do as the dentist asks, then your child will follow your example. Turn off your cell phone, and if you can, leave other children at school or with a sitter for the first visit.

What if my son starts crying or screaming?

Some children cry during a dental visit, especially the first visit, and most dental staff are comfortable handling upset children. If they cannot readily comfort your child, you may be asked to help calm him and reassure him that he is safe. It can be difficult to hear your child cry, but you know your child's cries best. If your little one is becoming hysterical, then you may need to insist that you provide a time-out for a quick hug and reassurance. Keep in mind that although you don't want your child to be terrified, his crying can actually help the dentist see inside his mouth better, so most of the time, dental staff can work around upset children. Your child's dentist may encourage you to reschedule the visit if it becomes too overwhelming. If this happens, ask the office staff for specific advice about what you can do differently next time to try to avoid problems.

Dental Tools and X-Rays

Mouth mirror. This is usually a small, round mirror at the end of a metal grip. The tool allows the dentist to examine a person's mouth from various directions. Sometimes this mirror has a light attached or magnifies the person's mouth and teeth for easier viewing.

Explorer. This is the metal hook-shaped pick that the dentist uses to check for cavities in teeth.

Periodontal probe. Also a metal hook, the probe measures the depth of the pocket in the gum and around the tooth to check for periodontal disease. The dentist can also use this probe to scrape beneath the gums to prevent plaque from hardening around the tooth.

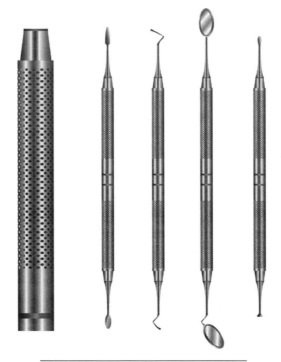

Dental instruments. © Len Neighbors / Photos.com

The bur. Commonly called the drill, this dental tool is often the most intimidating to patients. The bur is used to fill cavities and generally smooth out and polish teeth. Because this instrument can be painful, it is usually used with some type of numbing agent.

X-ray equipment. X-ray equipment varies from one dental office to another. All x-rays help detect any deep-lying problems in the teeth before they become visible to the human eye.

Cotton pliers. Cotton pliers look a lot like tweezers and function in the same way. They can be used to pick up small items and remove small items from the mouth. They also help avoid contamination.

Saliva ejector. A saliva ejector is a curved tube that acts as a vacuum inside the mouth to suction out saliva and other liquids. Since patients have to keep their mouths open for long periods at the dentist, saliva can become plentiful and interfere with the examination and treatment.

Will the staff use the actual names of the tools with my child?

Dental staff often use various phrases to describe what's happening in more kid-friendly language. Here are some of the terms your child may hear at the dentist:

- "Mr. Bumpy": an instrument that cleans out tooth decay slowly
- "Water whistle": an instrument that cleans out tooth decay quickly
- "Mr. Thirsty," "silly straw," or "tooth vacuum": the straw (saliva ejector) that removes water or saliva from the mouth
- "Sleepy juice": anesthetic that makes teeth feel tingly
- "Snugglie": protective stabilization to keep children safe
- "Sugar bugs": bacteria (germs) on the teeth
- "Tooth chair" or "Tooth pillow": tightly packed cotton rolls to help keep the mouth open or used in between teeth
- "Tooth pictures": x-rays
- "Tooth print": impression for an appliance, such as braces
- "Tooth raincoat and tooth ring": rubber square and ring that keep teeth dry
- "Tooth towel": gauze square
- "Tooth vitamins": fluoride treatment to keep teeth strong

> ### Words Matter
>
> Kids will live up (or down) to expectations, so talk to your child as if you expect her to have a good experience at the dentist. Don't use these words with your child when talking about the dentist:
>
> - Hurt
> - Shot
> - Pain
> - Sting
> - Pull
> - Drill
> - Poke
> - Needle
> - Yank
> - Cut
> - Pliers
> - Strap down
> - Tie up
> - Don't be scared
> - Are you scared?

How do dental offices clean and protect children against cross-contamination?

Several agencies set infection-control standards for all health care facilities, including dental practices. Involved agencies include the Joint Commission on Accreditation of Healthcare Organizations, the FDA, the

Centers for Disease Control and Prevention (CDC), the National Institute of Health, and the Occupational Safety and Health Administration (OSHA), as well as state agencies. Depending on their assigned roles, dental staff wear safety items such as gloves, masks, outer protective clothing, and protective eyewear or shields as appropriate. Experts agree that the chance of contracting an infectious disease during a routine visit is extremely rare. However, you should always feel free to ask about the office's sterilization process and their procedures for reducing the risk of cross-contamination.

Much of the office equipment, like air and water syringe tips, saliva ejectors, and high-speed suction tips, is disposable. Other instruments are cleaned after each use, using an ultrasonic scrubbing system, and then sterilized in an autoclave, a pressurized steam oven. One of the most important facets of operating a clean and safe practice is the frequency of staff hand washing.

Many offices post a list in their reception area or elsewhere of the infection-control procedures they follow. If you don't see this information, ask about it. Look around and see if the office looks clean and well cared for. If you see something that causes you concern, don't hesitate to ask questions.

Does Your Dental Practice Follow These Safety Guidelines?

To ensure the CDC and OSHA safety standards, the American Dental Hygienists' Association recommends that all dental offices:

- Use protective clothing, including gloves, masks, gowns or laboratory coats, and protective eyewear for all treatment procedures.
- Change gloves after each patient contact.
- Wash hands thoroughly before and after treating each patient.
- Heat-sterilize all nondisposable instruments and disinfect surfaces and equipment after treating each patient.
- Discard disposable needles, syringes, and other sharp instruments in puncture-resistant containers.
- Place all potentially infectious waste in closable, leak-proof containers or bags that are color-coded, labeled, or tagged in accordance with applicable federal, state, and local regulations.

What do dentists look for in x-rays?

Dental x-rays are diagnostic tools to allow dentists to diagnose problems accurately and treat dental conditions that might not be detected during a routine examination. X-rays can reveal problems such as damage to jawbones, impacted teeth, abscesses, cysts or tumors, and decay between the teeth. They are also important for recognizing cavities and erupting teeth as well as for diagnosing the effects of trauma and planning orthodontic treatment.

What types of x-rays are done on children's teeth?

A modern dental office uses machines that emit virtually no radiation—no more than your child would receive from a day in the sun or a weekend watching TV. As a precaution, however, your child should always wear a lead apron with a thyroid collar when having an x-ray.

Two main types of x-rays are used in dentistry: intra-oral (meaning the x-ray film goes in the mouth) and extra-oral (meaning the x-ray film is outside the mouth).

INTRA-ORAL X-RAYS

By far, intra-oral x-rays are the most common. They include several different types.

Bitewing x-rays show details of the upper and lower teeth in one area of the mouth. Each bitewing shows a tooth from its top to the bottom near the bone. These types of x-rays are used to detect decay between teeth and changes in bone density caused by gum disease. If the bitewing x-ray reveals cavities starting between the teeth, then the dentist can coach you and your child on better flossing techniques. These x-rays can also help with properly fitting a crown as well as determining the integrity of fillings.

Periapical x-rays show the entire tooth from the top to beyond the end of the root, where the tooth is anchored into the jaw. These x-rays are used to detect any abnormalities of the root structure and surrounding bone, including changes in the bone as a result of a tooth infection.

Occlusal x-rays are larger and show the full tooth development and placement. Each x-ray shows the entire arch of the teeth in either the upper or lower jaw.

EXTRA-ORAL X-RAYS

There are also several types of extra-oral x-rays, which use film outside the mouth.

Panoramic x-rays show the whole mouth—all the teeth in both the upper and lower jaws—on a single x-ray. For this, a special type of x-ray machine is used that moves around the head. Panoramic x-rays are useful for detecting the position of fully emerged teeth as well as emerging teeth. They can also help identify impacted teeth or diagnose tumors in the mouth.

Tomograms show a particular layer or slice of the mouth while blurring out all other layers. This type of x-ray helps point out structures that are difficult to see clearly because other structures are in the way.

Cephalometric projections show the entire side of the head as a profile picture, often as a way to see teeth in relation to the jaw. Orthodontists find this type of x-ray especially helpful.

Sialography uses a contrasting dye injection to see the salivary glands. This x-ray is typically used only if a problem with the salivary gland is suspected.

Computed tomography, also known as a CT scan, shows the body's interior structures as a 3-D image. CT scans for dental purposes are usually performed in hospitals to identify problems in the bones of the face, such as tumors or fractures. However, more and more dental offices now have their own CTs, also called cone

> ### How Safe Are Dental X-Rays?
>
> There is very little risk in dental x-rays. Dentists are keenly aware of the potential hazards of radiation exposure and recognize varying needs of each child based on risk factors. Lead aprons and high-speed film are used to ensure safety and minimize the amount of radiation. In addition, you are encouraged to bring x-rays from previous dentists to minimize unnecessary exposure. To put it into perspective, the risk of undiagnosed and untreated dental problems is far greater than the risk posed by radiation exposure from dental x-rays.

beam CTs. These are used most often by orthodontists. Oral surgeons also turn to CT scans to assess the quality and thickness of bone before placing implants, and endodontists use CT scans to complete root canal fillings.

How often do children's teeth need to be x-rayed?

As a general rule, children need x-rays more often than adults because a child's mouth grows and changes rapidly. Children are also more susceptible than adults to tooth decay. For children with a high risk of dental disease, the American Academy of Pediatric Dentistry recommends x-ray examinations every six months to detect cavities developing between the teeth. On average, most pediatric dentists request x-rays about once a year, especially for children with a low risk of tooth decay.

After the Appointment

What should I expect from the dentist at the end of the appointment?

The dentist should present you with an assessment of your child's oral health, instructions on oral home care, and information about the risks of cavities and, if relevant, finger, thumb, and pacifier habits. They may also provide you with information on dental growth and development and on preventing injury to the teeth and mouth. Expect to make your next dental appointment before you leave.

Digital X-Rays

Digital imaging is becoming more popular in dental offices, including those that treat children. Instead of developing an x-ray film in a dark room, the x-rays are sent directly from the machine to a computer. Images can then be viewed on a computer screen almost immediately, and they can be stored or printed out. There are many benefits to digital x-rays, particularly that digital imaging is easier and saves a lot of time. The images can be enhanced or enlarged, minimizing the need to take additional x rays. If necessary, the images can be easily sent to other dentists or specialists, and because the x-rays can be stored electronically, it is easy to compare images of certain teeth or changes even after many years. A disadvantage is that some digital sensors, which are placed in the mouth, are more bulky than film and may be difficult for a child to tolerate.

How long after the dental visit can my child eat or drink?

Normally, your child can eat or drink immediately following a dental visit. After a fluoride treatment, however, avoiding food or drink for the first 10 minutes can maximize the amount of fluoride available in the mouth during uptake. Although the fluoride sticks to the teeth immediately during a treatment, fluoride uptake in the enamel continues up to 12 hours. If you aren't sure exactly how long your child should hold off on eating or drinking after a dental visit, ask the dentist or other staff member before you leave the appointment.

How often should I take my child to the dentist?

If your child's teeth and gums are in good shape, you probably won't need to return for six months. If your child has a greater risk for oral health problems such as cavities, then she may need to see the dentist every three to four months. If further treatment is required, such as filling a cavity, you will need to come back for a follow-up appointment. Don't forget to ask the dentist any questions you have—this is your chance to get the answers you need.

CHAPTER 4 ▼

Preventing Decay and Protecting Teeth

Susan peered into her daughter's mouth as she brushed her teeth before bed. Even though she was dog-tired, she was faithful in making sure she always helped her 7-year-old brush and floss. Rebecca complied without complaining, used to her mom's diligent attention to her teeth. Susan knew how important it was to get her first grader to the dentist regularly, but she wasn't sure how long it had been since she'd made an appointment. Everything looked fine—with no dark spots anywhere. Susan made a mental note to make an appointment as soon as she had time.

Your child gets only two sets of teeth. That may seem like plenty, but once those secondary teeth come in during elementary school, they need to be healthy and strong enough to last for the next six or seven decades. Caregivers have a unique responsibility to make sure their child's choppers are in good condition into adulthood.

Protecting Your Child's Teeth

Protecting your child's teeth is a multipronged effort. Parents and caregivers must provide access to regular preventive dental care and treatment, brush and floss their children's teeth at least twice per day, provide tooth-healthy nutritional choices, and protect their children's teeth from injury. Protecting children's teeth also requires becoming fully informed about dental treatment options for children. For example, you will need to decide if fluoride and sealant treatments are appropriate.

Why Fluoride Is Important

Fluoride, a mineral that occurs naturally, makes the tooth's enamel more resistant to decay. Fluoride can be provided either systemically or topically. Fluoride in toothpaste, rinses, and applications at the dentist are all topical forms. Systemic fluoride is ingested, which allows it to be incorporated into the structure of tooth enamel as it forms. However, many believe topical fluoride is more effective because it aids in the remineralization (hardening) of enamel. Fluoridated water incorporates both systemic and topical contact and exposes children to very low levels of fluoride. Children who drink fluoridated water from birth experience up to 65 percent less tooth decay than those who don't.

Indirectly, fluoridation programs also help reduce the incidence of malocclusion, or improper bite, which can result in the premature loss of primary teeth or tooth structure. With fluoridation, there's less decay, which means fewer first teeth are lost prematurely. Children who brush regularly with fluoridated toothpaste have 24 percent fewer cavities than those who brush with nonfluoridated toothpaste.

Is fluoride safe?

The biggest risk with fluoride is fluorosis, when too much fluoride causes defects in the enamel of permanent teeth in children under 8 years of age. By age 8, the enamel of the permanent teeth has formed, and the risk of fluorosis is diminished. Fortunately, most cases are mild and will appear as tiny white specks or streaks that are often unnoticeable. In severe cases of enamel fluorosis, however, the appearance of the teeth is marred by discoloration or brown markings. The enamel may be pitted, rough, and hard to clean. Cosmetic dentistry can usually correct the appearance of such flaws, but the damage can't be reversed.

The best way to prevent fluorosis is to understand all the possible fluoride sources your child is exposed to and to discuss your child's risks with her dentist. Fluoride provides extraordinary benefits to children's teeth, and getting the right amount can protect your child's teeth for years to come. Still, there is a risk of toxicity from ingestion of too much fluoride, which is why toothpaste should be kept out of reach of young children and applied to the toothbrush by a parent.

What other sources of fluoride are there?

If you are concerned about the amount of fluoride your child may be consuming, talk to the dentist about your child's specific risks. The following foods and beverages may also contain fluoride.

Bottled water. Because the FDA does not require that fluoride content be listed on labels, it is difficult for consumers to know the fluoride content in their bottled water. If bottled water is your child's only source of water, you can probably assume she is receiving very low amounts of fluoride, if any.

Commercial beverages and foods. Many foods and beverages in stores and restaurants are made with community-fluoridated water. In addition, some foods naturally contain fluoride, such as seafood and some teas and fruit juices.

Infant nutrition. Human breast milk contains almost no fluoride. Even when the nursing mother drinks fluoridated water, the fluoride is not passed through the breast milk. Unless mixed with fluoridated water, powdered infant formula also contains little or no fluoride.

> *Do Water Filters Affect Fluoride Levels?*
>
> The fluoride content of fluoridated community water may be affected by water filters commonly used in homes. Most water filters use activated charcoal filters and cellulose filters, which do not really decrease fluoride content. Reverse osmosis filters, however, remove almost all fluoride from water. Distilled water does not contain any fluoride either.

Does my child need fluoride supplements?

Supplements should be considered for people whose community water source does not have fluoride and for children who are identified as being at high risk for developing tooth decay. Supplements are available in liquid, tablet, or lozenge form and aren't typically prescribed in children younger than 6 months of age. Don't add fluoride, however, without making sure your water sources do not have sufficient fluoride. Get a thumbs-up from your health care provider before supplementing your child's diet.

Does my child need fluoride treatments?

Professionally applied fluoride treatments are usually recommended twice per year. Fluoride treatments offer an average 21 percent reduction in decayed, missing, and filled tooth surfaces. Some dentists apply a fluoride varnish instead. A varnish is a professionally applied, sticky resin of highly concentrated fluoride. Typically, dental insurance dictates application frequency but not which type of fluoride is used. Many dental insurance agencies reimburse for fluoride once a year.

After the application of a fluoride varnish, your child will feel a coating over his teeth, and you may notice a difference in the color of your child's teeth while the varnish remains on them. To obtain the maximum benefit during the 4- to 6-hour treatment period, make sure your child follows these instructions after leaving the office:

- Do not eat or drink for 10 minutes following a fluoride varnish application.
- Do not remove the varnish by brushing or flossing for at least 4 to 6 hours.
- If possible, wait until tomorrow morning to resume normal brushing and flossing.
- Maintain a soft food diet during the treatment period.
- Avoid hot drinks and products containing alcohol, such as beverages, oral rinses, etc.

A thorough brushing and flossing the next day will easily remove any remaining varnish from your child's teeth. They will return to the same shine and brightness as before the treatment.

Does it matter if we have city or well water?

Fluoride has been added to public water systems since the 1940s, and fluoridated water has been hailed as one of the top ten greatest achievements in public health in the twentieth century. Chances are, if you have city water, you probably have fluoride. About 65 percent of the population in the United States now has access to optimally fluoridated water, defined as 0.7 parts per million (ppm).

How does your water compare? Although routine monitoring ensures appropriate fluoride levels, the U.S. Environmental Protection Agency (EPA) requires that all community water suppliers provide an annual report on the quality of water, including the fluoride concentration. Some post their annual reports on the EPA's Web site. You can also contact your local water authority directly for this information or find out the fluoride content of your town water by accessing the CDC Web site *My Water's Fluoride,* http://apps.nccd.cdc.gov/MWF/Index.asp.

If you have well water, be aware that wide variations in the natural fluoride concentration of well water sources exist. Private wells should be tested for fluoride concentration before fluoride supplements are taken. Testing can be done through local and state public health departments or private laboratories.

Do mouth rinses help prevent cavities?

Several different types of fluoride mouthwashes are available over-the-counter (without a prescription). Frequency of use ranges from daily to weekly. Schools used to have fluoride mouth-rinse programs, but most school systems have stopped using them because they are the least effective method for delivering fluoride to the teeth. Talk to your child's dentist about the use of fluoride-containing mouthwashes, especially if your child already uses fluoride toothpaste, drinks fluoridated water, and receives regular fluoride treatments. As with any type of dental mouthwash, fluoride rinses should only be used by children who can spit and won't swallow it.

Dental Sealants

Dental sealants may be one of the best-kept secrets in pediatric dentistry, with only one in four children having this cost-effective tooth defender on their molars. A plastic material applied to the chewing surface of permanent molars, dental sealants provide a physical barrier to bacterial invasion of pits and fissures. Some back teeth, especially molars, can be difficult for a person to clean because the grooves found on their chewing surface (the tooth's "pits and fissures") are deep and narrow. Even tooth brushing can't remove all the dental plaque because individual toothbrush bristles are too large to get into the depths of these teeth's grooves. When plaque isn't completely cleared away, these teeth are at risk of decay.

By bonding plastic resin, otherwise known as the dental sealant, into the grooves of a tooth, the dentist creates a smoother tooth surface. There aren't any areas left on the chewing surface of the tooth that the bristles of a toothbrush can't get to. Since dental plaque can be removed more effectively, there is less of a chance that tooth decay will form. Another difficulty associated with a tooth having deep grooves is that in some instances, the thickness of the enamel at the base of the grooves is thinner than the enamel that encases other aspects of the tooth. This means any decay that does form will have an easier time penetrating the enamel layer and will therefore progress more quickly into the inner parts of the tooth.

Sealants are effective because 90 percent of cavities in school-aged children occur in the pits and fissures of molars, the place a sealant covers. The first permanent molars erupt at age 6, and the second permanent molars around age 12, so these are the target ages for sealants, although they can be applied any time. For an individual tooth, a properly applied sealant is virtually 100 percent effective in preventing a cavity at the site of the sealant. Properly applied means applied when the tooth is dry and isolated, so that the sealant bonds to the enamel and grooves and

School-Based Sealant Programs

If you live in an area with a high percentage of students who receive free or reduced lunch, free sealant clinics may be offered at your child's school or community center. Check with your child's school nurse or guidance counselor to see if such services are available.

doesn't have an area of leakage. Sealants are only effective as long as they remain on the tooth.

Using sealants is a cost-effective strategy because they typically last five to ten years, and one sealant costs less than half that of a single filling. Sealants should be applied in all high-risk children around the ages of 6 and 12. They need to be used in addition to fluoride, because fluoride primarily benefits the smooth surfaces of teeth, whereas sealants protect the grooved surfaces.

Which teeth are best for sealants?

Permanent molars are the most likely to benefit from sealants. The sealant is most effective if applied soon after the teeth have erupted, before they have a chance to decay. Any tooth with deep grooves that place it at risk for tooth decay should be sealed. For example, if a child cannot easily clean a groove in a molar, then that groove needs a sealant. To identify teeth that need sealants, ask your child if any food feels caught on the tops of his back teeth that he can't fish out with his tongue. Sealants should be checked at your child's regular dental appointment and can be reapplied if they are no longer in place.

> *Allergy Alert*
>
> Dental sealants should not be given to children with an allergy to methacrylate. Methacrylate is contained in the sealant material, and the oral tissues may come in contact with it during sealant placement. Make sure your child's dentist office is aware of any allergies your child has.

How are sealants applied and how do they work?

Applying sealants is relatively simple and does not require drilling or disturbing the tooth. X-rays are usually performed first to make sure the sealants are not placed over existing tooth decay. Once those x-rays are completed, the process is quick and easy.

1. The tooth is cleaned.
2. The tooth is dried, and cotton is put around the tooth to keep it dry.
3. Because the sealant sticks better to a slightly rough surface, a solution is put on the tooth to roughen it.

4. The tooth is rinsed and dried again. Having a dry tooth is important so that the sealant will adhere well.

5. The liquid sealant is painted onto the tooth with a brush.

6. Finally, the dentist or dental hygienist shines a curing light on the tooth to help harden the sealant. In most cases, a blue light is emitted, which activates a catalyst in the sealant that initiates its set. It takes only about a minute for the sealant to form a protective shield around the tooth.

As with anything new placed in the mouth, your child may feel the sealant with her tongue. Sealants are very thin, however, and fill only the pits and grooves of molar teeth. The dentist will probably check how your child bites down on the sealed tooth to make sure that the sealant is not too thick. If it is, it can be buffed down. Your child can eat and drink immediately after the appointment with no problems or soreness. Dentists, dental hygienists, and certified dental assistants can all be trained to apply dental sealants to teeth.

Are sealants applied to baby teeth?

Some children have deep grooves in their baby teeth that would benefit from dental sealants. However, not all children need them on baby teeth. If you are concerned about whether your child needs sealants on primary teeth, speak to your child's dentist. It is unusual for dental insurance to cover sealants for these teeth.

Does my child need to brush as often with sealants?

Absolutely! Regular brushing and flossing is still critical even if you have sealants, especially between teeth where sealants aren't as effective. Although dental sealants help a lot in keeping teeth cavity-free, they should never replace good consistent oral care or eating healthy foods and visiting the dentist. All of this together will keep your child's teeth healthy and strong.

Are dental sealants safe?

For most children, dental sealants are a safe way to protect their teeth. Although the FDA is still investigating, it currently deems dental sealants safe. Some holistic dentists are cautious about using them, primarily because some, but not all, sealants contain bisphenol-A (BPA), or its chemical cousin bisphenol-A dimethacrylate (BPA-DMA). Sealants vary somewhat in their chemical makeup, and it is not clear how much exposure is damaging. Once the sealant is light cured, there is a trace amount of the uncured material (monomer) that can get into the system. The sealants do not leave BPA in the bloodstream in any measurable amounts, but sealant is left in the saliva for the first hour or so after application. The ADA recommends that dentists wipe off the surface of the cured sealant with a damp cotton pellet at the end of the procedure to remove this monomer. Discussing the pros and cons with your child's dentist could help you with your decision regarding sealants. If you decide to get the sealants for your child, find out the name of the product the dentist uses and do your research regarding the chemical content.

What Is a Holistic Dentist?

A holistic, or biological, dentist is one who approaches dentistry from an alternative, or complementary, perspective. Typically, holistic dentists do not recommend or place metal fillings, fluoride treatments, or sealants. They may also use hair analysis or recommend nutritional supplements or homeopathic remedies. The Holistic Dentistry Association offers a database of member dentists as well as additional information on the practice of holistic dentistry (www.holisticdental.org).

Who pays for sealants?

Although sealants can save money by preventing decay, they often cost as much as $60 a tooth. Your dental insurance may pay for part of the fees as a preventive measure, but may pay for sealants only on certain teeth. Your insurance company may not pay for reapplication if the sealant wears off before three years. If finances are a concern, talk to your child's dentist about putting sealants on the most vulnerable teeth and adding the others when you can afford them.

How Foods Affect Your Child's Teeth

Choosing healthy foods seems simple. Fruit and veggies are good, and candy is bad. Most parents have a good idea of what foods and beverages are good for their children's health. What they may not realize is the effect of their children's diet on their teeth. Children must have a balanced diet for their teeth to develop properly. They also need a balanced diet for healthy gum tissue around the teeth.

What are tooth-unfriendly foods?

Your child should stay away from sour candies—those promising a sweet and sour or "extreme sour" experience are very acidic. They can cause permanent erosion of the dental enamel on teeth and may lead to decay. If your child eats sour candy, suggest eating cheese or drinking milk afterward, or swishing with water, to neutralize the acids. Your child should then brush with fluoride toothpaste and a soft toothbrush.

We are used to thinking of candy as being bad for teeth, but we don't often think of foods like crackers and bread as being potentially damaging for teeth as well. Decay-causing bacteria thrive on carbohydrates; the acid they produce while a person is eating causes demineralization and leads to tooth decay.

Sticky foods like raisins and other dried fruit, cereal bars, gummies, and Fruit Roll-Ups are also bad for teeth, not only because they stick in the crevices and in between teeth, but because they are high in sugar. That doesn't mean you have to ban dried fruit or cereal bars from your child's diet, but

> **Xylitol**
>
> Xylitol is a low-calorie sugar substitute found in the fibers of many fruits and vegetables. Unlike other sweeteners, xylitol is beneficial for dental health. It has been shown to reduce tooth decay with regular use.

> **Medications, Sugar, and Tooth Decay**
>
> Many common children's medications contain sugar. Children are more likely to take sweet medicines without any fuss. Pay attention to medications in sugary liquids, especially if your child has to take them frequently. To cut down your child's risk for tooth decay, you can rinse out your child's mouth with water after giving medications that contain sugar; brush frequently if your child must take sugary medications multiple times a day; or speak to your pharmacist about sugar-free versions of the medications.

you do want to make sure your child brushes and flosses his teeth and regularly rinses his mouth out with water to prevent tooth decay.

What are tooth-friendly foods?

As hard as it is to get some children to eat, a healthy diet is important to healthy teeth. Some foods that tend to be better for teeth include cheeses and milk, which may contain properties that help prevent cavities, as well as vitamins and minerals that help with tooth development. Some researchers have suggested that chewing sugar-free gum containing xylitol after a meal can also help protect against cavities.

The American Academy of Pediatric Dentistry offers these suggestions regarding your child's diet and dental health:

The Cavity Count Checklist

The Palmer Classification rates various snacks based on their ability to produce cavities, according to research published in the Journal of the American Dental Association. The lower the number, the healthier the food is for your child's teeth.

Snack Item	Score
Peanut butter, nuts, vegetables	0
Cheese	1
Milk	2
Fruit juice, fresh fruit (excluding bananas)	3
Tortillas, pasta, rice, beans	4
Cereal	5
Crackers	6
Bread	7
Soda, Kool-Aid, other sweetened flavored drinks	8
Applesauce, yogurt, ice cream, pudding, Jell-O	9
Cookies, donuts, chips	10
Banana, raisins, jelly, jam	11
Candy	12

1. Ask your pediatric dentist to help you assess your child's diet.

2. Shop smart. Do not routinely stock your pantry with sugary or starchy snacks. Buy "fun foods" just for special times.

3. Limit the number of snack times, and choose nutritious snacks.

4. Provide a balanced diet, and save foods with sugar or starch for mealtimes.

5. Don't put your young child to bed with a bottle of milk, formula, juice, or soda. Limit the use of sippy cups with juice or soda between meals.

6. If your child chews gum or sips soda, choose products without sugar.

What should my child drink?

Fruit juices, milk, and sodas are common drinks of choice for children, but they can all do damage to growing teeth. The common denominator in all three? Sugar. In some ways, fruit juices are worse for teeth than a piece of chocolate. A cup of fruit juice, sipped throughout the morning, can literally coat your child's teeth in sugar for hours, causing teeth to decay more quickly. The best drink for children is simply water.

According to a study published in the *Archives of Disease in Childhood* (1995), more than 70 percent of preschool children never drink plain water. This alarming trend is influenced by a cultural shift toward juices and sugary or caffeinated drinks. Children imitate adults, including their preferences for sweeter drinks. Here's why water is so important for your child:

Healthy Halloween Handouts

Here are some tooth-healthy ideas for Halloween put together by the Minnesota Dental Association:

- sugarless gum
- stickers
- rubber spiders
- small packets of crayons or markers
- pencils with fun-shaped erasers
- small charms
- bags of trail mix or peanuts in the shell
- small chocolate candies (without caramel or components that will stick to teeth)

• Water makes up 80 percent of the brain and is essential for transmitting neurological signals.

• When we are thirsty, mental performance deteriorates by 10 percent.

• Being thirsty means we are already far behind in fluid intake. Feelings of thirst lag behind other physical symptoms.

Follow these steps to encourage your child to drink more water:

• Be a good role model. Drink water rather than sugar-based or caffeinated beverages such as juices and sodas.

• Offer and encourage water throughout the day. Keep pitchers of water or kid-sized water bottles in the refrigerator for the grab-and-go convenience of active children.

- Watch for signs of thirst and dehydration, including headache, lethargy, irritability, or inability to concentrate.

- Start early. Babies and toddlers can develop a preference for fruit juice, so get in the habit of offering water early in life.

Will extra vitamins protect my child's teeth?

Most children do not need additional vitamins because they get a variety of vitamins and minerals in a regular healthy diet. However, many parents prefer to offer a children's multivitamin as a kind of insurance against the occasional dietary mishap or a prolonged bout of picky eating.

Many multivitamins offer calcium, necessary for healthy bones and teeth. Children who drink milk and eat dairy products like yogurt and cheese usually get enough calcium from their diet without needing supplementation. Children who have milk allergies or who just don't like milk may need help meeting their calcium requirements through other foods, such as calcium-fortified orange juice. Vitamins, even those with extra calcium, generally have only about 200 mg of the mineral, or 20 percent of daily requirements, so you need to supplement with other high-calcium foods anyway. Vitamin D is also important, as it promotes bone and tooth formation and helps the body absorb calcium. Good sources of vitamin D include milk, cheese, and yogurt (especially fortified dairy products), egg yolks, and fish oil. Being out in the sun for about 10 minutes a day also boosts vitamin D levels.

How Much Juice Does My Child Need?

The American Academy of Pediatrics reminds parents that children do not need fruit juice to be healthy. Although 4 to 6 ounces of fruit juice is roughly equivalent to a serving of fruit, it doesn't offer the same benefits as fruit. If you do offer fruit juice to your children, limit it to 6 ounces a day. Most fruit juices can also be watered down with little difference in taste.

Can Vitamins Hurt My Child's Teeth?

Although vitamins may contain ingredients that help build strong teeth, they can also contribute to tooth decay. Some vitamins, especially those designed for children, contain sugar. If the vitamins are soft and gummy, that sugar might stick to the surfaces of teeth and in between teeth for hours before being brushed away. If your child takes a gummy-type vitamin, make sure she brushes and flosses her teeth soon afterward. Better yet, find a different source for the vitamins.

Is chewing gum okay for teeth?

Chewing gum in moderation is fine if it is sugar-free. In fact, chewing gum contributes to plaque reduction, and some studies have shown beneficial effects on oral hygiene, calculus, and gingivitis. In fact, people who chew sugar-free gum with xylitol three times a day reduce their risk of tooth decay by 40 percent compared with those who do not chew gum.

It is best to chew soon after eating. Chewing for about 15 minutes removes food debris and plaque and stimulates the flow of saliva. Sugar-free chewing gum is also recommended for people with xerostomia (dry mouth) to increase saliva, along with drinking more water (six to eight glasses a day). Children who experience TMJ (temporomandibular joint) disorder should refrain from any gum chewing.

> *Who Invented Chewing Gum?*
>
> William F. Semple, an Ohio dentist, used rubber to create a product for jaw exercise and gum stimulation. He received the first patent to manufacture chewing gum in December 1869.

Is xylitol good for teeth?

Xylitol is a sweet substance commonly found in birch trees and in the fibrous portions of many fruits and vegetables. Originally approved as an artificial sweetener especially helpful for people who have diabetes, it has gained worldwide attention in promoting better dental health. Xylitol inhibits the ability of cavity-causing bacteria (mainly *Streptococcus mutans*) in your mouth to adhere to the surfaces of your teeth. In turn, this prevents the bacteria from forming dental plaque. Xylitol also reduces the acid-producing potential of the bacteria, lessening the chance of tooth decay. Although it shouldn't replace brushing and flossing, adding xylitol gum to your child's daily habits may prove to be just what the dentist ordered.

How much xylitol does my child need?

While products containing xylitol are good for teeth, not all products have the same amount of it. When you read the ingredients list, look for

---

Homemade Xylitol Mouthwash

If you are ambitious, you can harness the power of xylitol with a simple mouthwash recipe. You'll need to make a trip to your local health food store for the ingredients, but once you get them, it's easy to make. Add 1 teaspoon of pure xylitol, 1/4 teaspoon of sea salt, and 1/4 teaspoon of calcium lactate. If you can't find calcium lactate, you can use calcium carbonate, otherwise known as baking soda. Put these three ingredients in a glass and add enough hot water to cover them. Stir to dissolve the powders. After it's a comfortable temperature, rinse and gargle with the mixture.

The longer the exposure to your teeth and gums, the better. If possible, try to do this at least a few times a day. This is only for older children who can swish and spit without swallowing. Xylitol is toxic for dogs, so don't leave it around for Fido to drink.

---

xylitol to be listed first. If cheaper sweeteners like mannitol or sorbitol are listed as second or third ingredients, it may indicate a lower level of xylitol. Be careful when comparing the labeling found on different gums. Their xylitol content may be stated in terms of serving size. In the case of chewing gum products, you may find that a single serving size is either one or possibly two sticks of gum.

For small children, consuming 5 to 6 grams of xylitol each day (divided up into three to five doses spread throughout the day) is appropriate, while teens and adults should use 6 to 10 grams per day, divided up into three to five doses for maximum cavity-busting properties.

CHAPTER 5

Affording Dental Care for Your Child

"Thanks so much for coming in today, Mrs. Ledger." The receptionist handed her a brightly colored piece of paper, explaining, "This is the estimate after insurance for the fillings that Dr. Cooper talked to you about. Would you like to go ahead and make an appointment?" Karen blinked, trying to mentally calculate when she would have an "extra" two hundred dollars. "Let me check my work calendar and get back with you," she answered, wondering how two such tiny teeth could be so expensive.

Taking care of your child's teeth can get pricey. Although toothpaste is relatively inexpensive, fillings aren't. Some families have dental insurance, but about half of Americans have to pay 100 percent of their dental care costs. On average, Americans spend $315 per person annually on dental care, totaling over $95 billion a year. For a family with several children, paying for dental visits can add up quickly.

Keeping teeth and gums healthy by practicing good oral hygiene and seeing the dentist regularly can help your child avoid more serious oral health problems and more extensive—and expensive—treatment. When children see a dentist more often, less extensive dental care is likely to be needed. Seventy percent of children treated for

The Most Expensive Tooth

You think your children's teeth are expensive? Consider this—John Lennon's tooth sold at auction for $31,000. He had given it to his housekeeper, who gave it to her niece for a souvenir. The buyer, a Canadian dentist, didn't say why he wanted the tooth.

serious dental problems before age 5 have never been examined by a dentist before. Not taking your child to the dentist early on can eventually cost you thousands of dollars.

Dental Insurance

Although dental insurance isn't perfect, it offers benefits. The most important one? People with dental insurance are more likely to visit the dentist for regular preventive treatment. Routine exams allow a dentist to get to know patients and follow their health history. Dentists are better able to catch and treat potential problems early when they see their patients routinely. If you have dental insurance, your entire family's teeth are likely to be healthier.

Dental insurance plans are designed to help cover the costs employees experience in obtaining necessary dental care. Dental insurance plans generally cover $1,000 to $1,350 in dental care costs annually. A dental insurance plan may cover the following care, at different percentages, depending on the plan:

> **Does Dental Insurance Really Make a Difference?**
>
> Overall, 42 percent of people have a dental visit each year, regardless of how many people have insurance coverage. People with private dental insurance, however, were more than three times more likely to have a dental visit than those without dental insurance. If you are undecided about buying dental insurance, talk to your dentist about the plan you're considering and if it is appropriate for your family's treatment.

- Diagnostic and preventive care
- Periodontal maintenance and cleanings
- Basic restorative treatment, such as fillings
- Oral surgery, such as pulling a tooth
- Root canals
- Orthodontics (braces): usually not covered or covered with a set fee as a one-time benefit that is only a small portion of the total cost

Each family's needs and available insurance options vary. Another advantage of having dental insurance is discounted fees for services, although you need to read the fine print. Know what the annual limits are and if there is a waiting period for extensive work. Dental insurance companies limit their liability (that is, how much they will pay out) in part by limiting the amount of a dentist's fee that they deem acceptable. This limit has been called the "usual and customary" fee. Their contract stipulates that the company will pay a certain percentage, say 50 or 80 percent, of the "usual and customary" charges for a particular procedure.

Setting a "usual and customary" charge is reasonable for an insurance plan to do. Medical, homeowners', and auto insurance all have similar provisions. The insurance company does this to protect itself against possible price gouging. It can't guarantee payment of any fee that service providers may charge. If your dental insurance company is supposed to pay 100 percent of usual and customary fees for a filling, for example, and your dentist charges $25 more than the usual and customary fee, then that $25 is your responsibility. You can, however, research what other dentists in the area charge for the same service; if you find that other dentists charge the same as or more than your dentist charges, you can petition your dental insurer to reevaluate its usual and customary rate.

> *In or out of Network?*
>
> Most dental plans use a network of participating dentists in your area. This means that the plan will reimburse bills received only from a specified list of dental providers (of usual and customary fees). Some dentists will be in your network, and some won't be. Before you sign up for the dental plan, research the providers on the list. Are their offices close enough to you to be convenient? Are there pediatric dentists on the list? Is it worth changing dentists if you have already established a good relationship with one?

What if I don't have dental insurance for my child?

The *Journal of the American Dental Association* (2012) reports that 77 percent of children in the United States have dental insurance. Of these, 29 percent have public dental insurance, such as Medicaid. Overall, according to this study, 16.3 million children lack dental insurance, 2.6 times the number of children who do not have medical insurance. Children who are uninsured for dental care are less than half as likely to receive preventive dental care. African American children, insured or not, are significantly less likely than white children to receive preventive dental care.

You don't need dental insurance to receive dental care for your child. Although most physicians require their patients to have health insurance, dental offices rarely exclude self-pay patients. Dental insurance is probably a wise financial move if you are currently living on a strict household budget with little or no money in savings. If your child has a broken tooth or other major dental calamity, paying $1,500 for a dental procedure will make your financial situation even tighter.

Where can I get dental insurance?

Some employers offer dental insurance policies for their staff. They may pay for all or a portion of the cost. The employee's fees are usually paid through a payroll deduction. Some employers do not pay for dental insurance, but employees may purchase insurance in a company dental insurance plan at a discounted price.

If your company does not offer such an option, you may be eligible for a plan if you belong to an organization such as a local business group, college alumni association, or fraternal association. Check the membership information online to see if the group provides access to a group dental insurance plan. Some plans are offered online, but options are limited. Instead, look for an insurance broker who has good connections to insurance companies. A broker can help you to find a reputable company that offers affordable dental insurance plans.

When both parents have dental coverage options, they may have to choose between dental plans. If this is your situation, carefully evaluate the benefits you will be eligible for under each plan. States set guidelines regulating coordination of benefits, which means that when a patient is covered under more than one group dental plan, benefits paid by all plans will be limited to 100 percent of the actual charges after each deductible has been satisfied. If both you and your partner have dental plans, the insurance companies may set rules that dictate which insurance is primary. Some policies are gender based, indicating, for example, that the father's insurance is always primary, while other companies set more arbitrary rules, such as which parent's birthday is first in the calendar year.

Many companies allow employees to sign up or change dental coverage within a month of the hire date and then one month each year, during open enrollment. You may have several different dental plans to choose from. Don't assume the plan you've always chosen is the best one. Before making your choice each year, ask a representative of the insurance company to supply you with a copy of the benefits handbook, where you will find detailed patient information about the coverage and its limitations and exclusions. Familiarize yourself with the plan's provisions, and if you have questions about the coverage or calculation of benefits or any other important point, ask an insurance company representative before you make a decision.

When you are choosing among dental insurance plans, consider these questions:

- Can you choose your own dentist? Some dental insurance plans will restrict you to certain dentists, while others allow you to choose.
- Who decides on the best treatment for your child? Some dental insurance plans restrict payment to the least expensive treatment, even though there may be other, more effective, treatment options.
- What is covered? A solid dental insurance plan should cover two cleanings a year with either a small office visit fee or no fee. X-rays and fluoride treatments are also usually covered at no additional cost. The fees for other services are usually split 50/50 between the insurance plan and the patient, up to the plan's maximum payout amount depending on the policy. Less coverage costs less.
- Will you be limited to certain times for appointments? Some dentists limit scheduling times for particular dental insurance participants.
- What will you pay? What are the specific costs for services with this plan?

What are limitations and exclusions?

As with any insurance plan, most dental plans include limitations and exclusions. Pay special attention to exclusion and limitation clauses and find out about the services not covered by the policy when it first goes into effect. The two most common causes—a missing tooth clause and a replacement clause—mean that no dental treatment will be covered by the insurance company for teeth lost before the policy went into effect. Another important clause in some policies requires a waiting period from the time the insurance coverage begins until you are given complete coverage.

Is dental insurance worth the expense?

The monthly premiums depend on the number of people in your family who need coverage, the insurance company, your location, and the plan you choose. For example, if the monthly premium per person averages $50 a month, then you are spending $600 on dental costs each year per person, even if a family member doesn't get any dental work done beyond the twice-a-year cleaning and exam. Only you can decide if it's worth it. Routine dental care of two visits a year probably won't add up to more than $600, but add in a couple of cavities or a broken tooth, and you'll be glad you have insurance.

Why doesn't our dentist accept our dental insurance?

From the dental office's perspective, a good insurance company pays what it states it will pay in a timely manner without insisting on unnecessary paperwork. An insurance company has a legal obligation to pay what is written in the contract, but sometimes it can be hard to collect. Dentists judge an insurance company by how well it fulfills its obligations to its policyholders and how much trouble the office has to go through to collect payment. If it involves too much trouble, then it isn't cost effective for the dental practice to accept that particular insurance carrier, so it won't.

Some dentists simply refuse to accept dental insurance at all. They have decided that the price they have to charge to cover the cost of doing the insurance paperwork is simply too high. Typically, such dentists have lower fees because they have lower overhead. This isn't always the case, so you'll want to do your homework first.

Understanding Billing

When you see a traditional health care provider, whether in the hospital or in a private practice,
your bill is usually divided into services, with each
service accompanied by a number. That number is
a code for the insurance company's billing department. If your insurance pays on that particular
code, it reimburses at the agreed-on rate. Your
dental insurance is the same way. Dental services are billed using Current Dental Terminology
(CDT-5), a code set with descriptive terms developed and updated by the American Dental Association (ADA) for reporting dental services and
procedures to dental benefits plans.

How do I get reimbursed for my dental expenses?

This is one of the first questions you will want
to ask when you make an appointment. Each doctor's office handles billing and financial arrange-
ments differently. Some dentist's offices bill your
insurance and ask you to pay the copay at the time of service. Other dental
offices require you to pay 100 percent of the visit and then you have to file
the paperwork yourself to get reimbursed. Whether the office will file for
you may depend on the type of insurance you have. Even if an office is less
expensive because you have to file the paperwork, factor in the hassle and
the possibility of not getting the paperwork done. If you are well organized, then the extra headache may be worth the savings.

Even with dental insurance, why do I still have a huge bill?

If we go to the hospital for a medical problem, we expect the initial
bill to be an outrageous sum, but we shrug it off, knowing that the health

---

Common CDT Codes for Dental Exams

- D0120 periodic oral evaluation: established patient
- D0140 limited oral evaluation: problem focused
- D0145 oral evaluation for
a patient under 3 years of
age and counseling with
primary caregiver
- D0150 comprehensive
oral evaluation: new or
established patient
- D0160 detailed and extensive oral evaluation: problem focused, by report
- D0170 re-evaluation:
limited, problem focused
(established patient, not
postoperative visit)
- D0180 comprehensive
periodontal evaluation:
new or established patient

insurance company will work its magic, and somehow the "real" bill we pay will be more manageable. We don't usually have the same experience with our dental insurance. Instead, we get the total, often having to pay up front, and we start to wonder what good dental insurance does anyway. Those expectations are part of the problem. Dental insurance is not designed to act like health insurance. In other words, not everything is covered. Instead, dental insurance is primarily a preventive benefit that provides limited assistance when more complicated work is required.

Why won't the dentist's office bill me?

Most dental offices do not bill or extend credit. They expect full payment at each visit for services provided. If you have dental insurance, the front office will often confirm what your insurance company will pay and let you know what your estimated payment will be. Should insurance pay an amount different from what the office anticipates, the dental office will usually bill you the difference. Otherwise, dental offices usually accept cash, checks, or credit cards and may offer in-house or out-of-house finance programs. If you need to borrow money to pay for the dentist, shop around; your bank may be able to offer you a better deal on a loan than the credit agency your dentist recommends.

You Can Take It with You

If you move and need to change dentists, get copies of your family's dental records to take to the new dentist. Otherwise, additional diagnostic testing may need to be done. You may have to pay a small fee to have your child's records copied, and you will usually have to sign a Release of Information form, giving permission for your child's records to be sent to a new practice.

What is a pretreatment estimate?

You should get a pretreatment estimate from the dentist before you agree to any treatments. The estimate lets you know up front exactly what the procedure entails, how long it will take, how much things will cost, what your insurance plan will pay, and the amount for which you will be responsible. It also gives you the opportunity to discuss with your child's dentist any alternatives that will lower your costs while still meeting your child's dental care needs. A pretreatment estimate is always a good idea to avoid surprises later, especially if you are considering more costly procedures, such as crowns or tooth extractions.

Unfortunately, the pretreatment estimate has its limitations. The most important one is that it is only a guide to potential payment and not a legally binding contract. After all, a lot can happen before and during treatment. Your tooth could be further damaged, requiring additional treatments. Benefits may have been exhausted since the approval was granted, or the insurance policy may have changed. Even if the estimate clearly states that a procedure will be covered, you may later learn that the promised benefit will be only partially paid or not paid after all. Although this is rare, it does happen. When it does, you are still obligated to pay the entire bill. Be sure to familiarize yourself with the most current benefits package and updates and get the insurance company's estimate in writing. In addition, try to avoid a large time gap between when the estimate is given and when the dental work is done. Know how long the estimate is good for. If too much time elapses, get a new estimate.

> **What Is a Treatment Plan?**
>
> Your estimated bill is based on the treatment plan created by your dentist. The dentist will mark teeth using a chart that numbers each tooth based on the Universal Numbering System. The markings are spots where decay is noted or has already been treated. Work that needs to be done is indicated with red ink, while work that is completed is marked in blue. The treatment plan should include a description of what will be done for each tooth; if necessary for successful treatment, comfort, or finances, the work can be done over the course of several different visits.

Other Ways to Pay for Dental Care

What are dental discount plans?

Dental discount plans can be an attractive alternative to costly dental insurance without the hassle of deductibles or claim forms. Here's how they work: you pay an annual fee, usually somewhere between $100 and $300, and then you receive 10 percent to 60 percent off the cost of care at participating dental providers. What's the catch? The plans don't always work out, for various reasons. Do your homework. Ask around and see if you personally know anyone who has used the plan you are considering.

Before you buy, ask for a list of participating dentists in your area. Call those dentists to confirm the relationship and the discount.

Can I finance dental care for my family?

What can you do when you simply can't pay for the dental work your child needs? Several companies offer credit card–type programs specifically for health care. If you pay on time, some of the companies will allow a no-interest repayment option for several months. The caveat is that if minimum monthly payments are not met, interest charges accrue at a variable rate that's currently about 23 percent. It's not ideal, but it is cheaper than putting the charge on most credit cards.

Your dentist's office will likely have information about getting a loan for dental care. However, among the different companies that offer such services, the one your dental office uses may not be the best one for you. Shop around before you sign this loan. To get a loan, most companies require government identification and a current checking account with printed checks.

Does regular medical insurance ever cover dental expenses?

Medical insurance rarely covers dental work. (Most medical insurance lists exclusions in the paperwork it sends to participants and prospective participants.) Many medical insurance companies, however, will cover at least a portion of the fees for oral surgery, especially if it is done under general anesthesia. For example, medical insurance may pay for impacted wisdom teeth removal. If you're unsure, contact your company's benefits representative for more information. Possibly both dental and medical insurance policies will pay a portion of the bill.

Are dental bills tax deductible?

According to IRS publication 502, you can include in medical expenses the amounts you pay for the prevention and treatment of dental disease. Preventive treatment includes the services of a dental hygienist or dentist for such procedures as teeth cleaning, the application of sealants, and fluoride treatments to prevent tooth decay. Treatment to alleviate dental disease includes services of a dentist for procedures such as x-rays, fillings, braces, extractions, dentures, and other dental ailments. Cosmetic dentistry, such as tooth whitening, is not covered.

Can I negotiate rates with my dentist?

In 2006, *Money Magazine* reported that a national survey found that 10 percent of respondents had haggled with their dentists over fees, and 64 percent had been successful in getting a price break. It's perfectly appropriate to talk to your dentist about payment options. Explain to the dentist that you want to use him to perform the dental work you need done, but the fee is outside your price range. Asking if the rates can be lowered may lead to a reduced fee. Be polite and reasonable. The average negotiated rate is a 10 percent deduction. Ask the office staff if they offer a discount for paying by cash or check rather than credit card.

Are there other ways to save money at the dentist?

If your child needs to have work done—especially expensive treatments—get a second opinion. When you do, make sure the financial billers at both offices run the numbers with your insurance company so you can compare apples to apples. For major work, a second opinion is critical because the differences in fees can be hundreds of dollars. If you'd prefer to use the dentist with the higher rate, ask that dentist to match the written estimate of the other dentist.

What if I can't afford to take my child to the dentist?

If you do not have health insurance and you cannot afford the dental visit fees, you may still be able to get dental care for your children. Most states have a dental association that maintains a list of clinics and special programs that provide dental services to patients who are on public care programs or that offer services at a reduced cost. Check online for the dental agency in your state. Do not assume that your children will have to go without dental care. With some research, you may be able to locate free or affordable dental services for your children.

FEDERAL PROGRAMS

Medicaid is the largest source of funding for medical, dental, and other health-related services for people with limited incomes. More than 40 million people have Medicaid coverage, about half of them children. To be approved to receive the funding, you must meet certain eligibility requirements. Go to http://cms.hhs.gov to look up the requirements in your state.

STATE DENTAL COVERAGE

Each state in the United States has a health and dental program for children who come from low-income families. Under the Children's Health Insurance Plan (CHIP), each qualified child whose family income is under its income requirement bracket is either covered for free or is given low-cost insurance. However, dental appliances, such as braces or sports-related mouth protection, other orthodontic costs, and cosmetic dentistry are not covered by CHIP. For more information, contact your state's health department.

I have Medicaid, but it's hard to use. What do I do?

If your child is on Medicaid, his dental care is covered until age 21. That does not mean, however, that it will be easy to find a dentist to accept Medicaid as a form of payment. Some dentists will not accept it because the reimbursement amounts are so low, sometimes even costing the dentist to treat patients. Additionally, for reasons often beyond their control, Medicaid patients are more likely to skip scheduled appointments, and many dentists enforce a limit of one or two skipped appointments before refusing to see the patient again.

If your child is on Medicaid and you cannot locate a dentist in your area, contact your local health department, your child's school counselor, or your social worker for suggestions. You may also have a caseworker assigned to you who can help you locate service providers.

Are there other resources for low-cost or free dental care?

Go back to school—dental school, that is. At most dental schools, you and your child can receive low-cost dental treatment delivered by supervised dental students. Services offered typically include examinations, x-rays, teeth cleaning, fluoride treatments, fillings, extractions, and emergency pain relief. Patients are treated by third-year and fourth-year students; every step of a dental procedure done by a student must be inspected and checked off by a teacher, who is an experienced and licensed dentist. Many dental schools and hospitals also have pediatric dentistry residency programs, where dental graduates are training to be pediatric dentists. The fees are usually less than for dentists in practice, and the services include all the things previously mentioned as well as treatment under sedation or general anesthesia. Dental hygiene schools are another resource for low-cost preventive care.

Your local health department is also a good source for information on available services in your area. Many school systems have social workers or counselors on staff who are aware of cost-effective care and mobile dental services. In addition, your state's dental association can be an excellent resource. Free dental screenings and dental care are often offered during Children's Dental Health Month in February, when thousands of the nation's dentists and their dental team members provide free oral health care services to children from low-income families across the country. In fact, many states sponsor an annual Mission of Mercy event, where children and adults can receive free care. To find dental programs targeting underserved children near you, contact the American Dental Association (www.ada.org) or America's ToothFairy (www.ncohf.org).

PART II

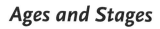

Ages and Stages

CHAPTER 6 ▼

Pregnancy and Your Baby's Teeth

When Sarah found out she was pregnant, she did everything by the book. She ate well, took her prenatal vitamins, avoided secondhand smoke, and wore her seatbelt everywhere. She was the picture of pregnant health. What she didn't do was go to the dentist. Her teeth looked and felt fine, and she was not a big fan of the dentist, so it was an easy appointment to "forget" to make. She didn't realize that good oral care for a child starts before birth.

Sarah's not alone. Only about one-third of pregnant women visit the dentist while they are pregnant. Worse yet, only half of pregnant women who report having a dental problem get dental care. With very few exceptions, routine dental examinations or treatment should be performed on schedule during pregnancy. In fact, not going to the dentist may cause such problems as oral infections that can affect the fetus or create the need for emergency care.

Get regular checkups and cleanings during pregnancy to keep your mouth as healthy as possible. Research proves that prevention, diagnosis, and treatment of oral diseases, including limited dental x-rays, if needed, and the use of local anesthesia, can be undertaken during pregnancy with very little risk to mom or baby compared with the risk of not getting dental care.

When to Get Dental Care

If your pregnancy was planned, then in an ideal world, you had any dental problems taken care of during your preconception planning. If so, good for you! It is ideal to get x-rays and dental work taken care of before a pregnancy so that you and baby get off to a good start.

Here is something else to consider: regular dental checkups may help protect your fertility. If you're ready to grow your family, and it isn't happening, check to see if you're due for a dental visit. The inflammation from gum disease can delay conception for several months. Such inflammation is also thought to be linked to repeat miscarriages, failed IVF treatments, and decreased chances for pregnancy in women over age 40. Be aware that taking ovulation-inducing drugs during fertility treatments has a side effect of putting moms-to-be at greater risk for gingivitis.

> **Male Fertility and Oral Health**
>
> Dad's oral health matters too. Research published in the *Journal of Clinical Periodontology* in 2011 found an association between gum disease and male fertility. Many men with gingivitis and periodontitis also had low sperm counts and diminished semen quality.

What if I don't visit the dentist? My teeth seem healthy enough.

Many studies have shown that women who have a preterm delivery are more likely to have had gum disease during pregnancy. (Chapter 13 discusses gum disease in detail.) This makes sense, because gum disease is a bacterial infection, and infections in any area of the body can cause preterm labor and delivery. Disease-causing bacteria produce toxins that pass into the bloodstream. This may cause the body to produce other chemicals to try to fight off the infection, the same chemicals that can induce contractions or preterm labor. Pregnant women who receive treatment to prevent gum disease are less likely to have a preterm baby than women who have untreated gum disease.

> **Gingivitis and Pregnancy**
>
> Gingivitis, the mildest form of gum disease, is experienced by 60 to 75 percent of all women and is the most common oral condition in pregnancy. All women need to pay attention to oral health to prevent long-term problems.

What dental care can I receive during pregnancy?

Be sure to tell all your health care providers that you are pregnant, because pregnancy may affect your treatment plan. The key to dental care during pregnancy is not to neglect your six-month checkups—they are vital to maintaining a healthy mouth. Changes in hormone levels during pregnancy can increase tooth sensitivity and gum bleeding, so you may experience slight bleeding during dental checkups even if you normally don't. Avoid elective dental treatment, such as routine dental x-rays, bonding, and teeth whitening, especially during the first trimester. Research is unclear regarding sealant use in pregnancy. It's probably better to play it safe and wait until after baby arrives before adding a sealant.

Although some dental procedures should be done when you aren't pregnant, a dental emergency may require treatment. When does the risk outweigh the benefit? Consider treatment if it is necessary to relieve pain, prevent an infection, or decrease stress on you or your fetus. Before you have anything beyond routine care performed, contact your primary health care provider, obstetrician, or midwife.

X-rays should be limited but are acceptable if they are necessary. Radiation from dental x-rays is extremely low, but every precaution should be taken to minimize radiation exposure. A lead apron is used to minimize exposure to the abdomen, and a leaded thyroid collar should be used to protect the thyroid from radiation. When both a lead apron and a thyroid shield are appropriately used, pregnant women do not need to worry if x-rays are needed to provide appropriate dental care.

Although your dentist may have experience in treating pregnant women, your obstetrician or midwife is a more expert resource about what's

> **Will My Medical Insurance Pay for My Dental Care?**
>
> This varies greatly depending on the insurance plan. The best advice is to make sure you ask. Many people assume it won't pay anything, so they never ask—and their failure to ask ends up costing them more out of pocket. Even when a health insurance company does not pay for routine dental care, some progressive medical insurers recognize that a pregnant woman's dental care can affect her unborn baby's health. As a result, a coordination of benefits may be possible for some pregnant women. Contact your health insurance company to see if dental coverage might be available.

safe for you and baby. If you're not sure about a procedure, wait until you can get clearance from your health care provider. This is especially true if you need anesthetic for a dental procedure.

Can I take medications my dentist prescribes?

Most drugs commonly used in dentistry are considered safe to use during pregnancy. The FDA requires manufacturers to label all medications with one of five pregnancy medication categories as a way to classify the risk of taking each medication during pregnancy. Although no medication is completely safe, the classifications provide a way for pregnant patients and health care providers to make educated decisions about whether to use a particular drug. Before taking any medication your dentist recommends, even an over-the-counter medicine, talk to your primary health care provider or obstetrician.

Relieving pain and fever are important during pregnancy. Untreated fever can cause problems with the baby's development, especially during the first trimester. Severe pain can cause intense stress on the body, leading to high levels of stress hormones and increased blood pressure, neither of which is good for your developing baby. Acetaminophen (Tylenol) is usually recommended for pain relief because aspirin and nonsteroidal anti-inflammatory drugs, like ibuprofen (e.g., Motrin or Advil), can cause bleeding or other complications. You should never take any drugs in the tetracycline family during pregnancy because they can cause damage to the baby's developing teeth. Before taking any medications, talk to your health care provider.

> *Should I Take Fluoride Supplements to Help Baby's Growing Teeth?*
>
> Pregnant women do not need fluoride supplements for their growing babies. Current evidence suggests there is little to no benefit to baby's teeth when pregnant women take fluoride supplements. Instead, focus on maintaining your own healthy smile.

How Pregnancy Affects Your Teeth

How do I help my bleeding gums?

You may notice an increase in gum tenderness during pregnancy, and this is perfectly normal. Regular periodontal, or gum, examinations are critical during pregnancy, because hormonal changes put you at a higher risk for periodontal disease and for tender gums that bleed easily—also known as pregnancy gingivitis. In addition to brushing and flossing, using alcohol-free mouthwash each night after brushing and flossing may help cut down on bacteria and help gums heal.

My dentist said I have pregnancy tumors on my gums. Should I be worried?

Pregnancy tumors sound worse than they are. Officially known as *pyogenic granuloma,* they can be located anywhere on the body and have absolutely nothing to do with cancer. In the mouth they are simply non-cancerous tissue growths that develop when swollen gums become irritated and inflamed. Usually these tumors shrink after the pregnancy is over. If they remain on the gums after pregnancy, they may need to be removed by a periodontist or oral surgeon.

My grandmother swears she lost a tooth with every child. Will pregnancy ruin my teeth?

While it might have been true for your grandmother, it doesn't have to be true for you. There is no reason for a healthy woman receiving regular dental care to lose any teeth—even during a pregnancy. The underlying myth behind "gain a child and lose a tooth" is that the baby needs calcium, so it is leached from the mother's teeth during pregnancy. Not true. The calcium your baby needs comes from your diet, not your choppers. If you notice your teeth becoming loose or other unusual signs, call for an urgent dental appointment. It is true, though, that the more children a woman has, the more likely she is to have dental problems. Researchers suspect the reason is that moms are more likely than women without children to snack on sugary kid foods.

Does morning sickness affect my teeth?

For some women, morning sickness lasts just a few weeks; for others, it lasts the entire pregnancy. Morning sickness affects more than the tummy. It can cause problems with oral health if the nausea makes it difficult to use a toothbrush or floss. Some women are so sensitive to gagging while pregnant that they have a hard time tolerating anything placed in the mouth. If nausea disrupts routine brushing and flossing, then the bacteria normally present in the mouth are likely to cause pregnancy gingivitis or tooth decay.

Nausea and vomiting often go together, especially during the first trimester. During the third trimester, some women develop severe heartburn or esophageal reflux, which propels stomach acid up into the mouth. Stomach acids irritate the gingival tissue. Stomach acids also dissolve tooth enamel and soften the outer layers of the tooth. This process is called dental erosion. The enamel will be thinned if it repeatedly comes into contact with these acids.

Brushing during Pregnancy

Many pregnant women have trouble brushing their teeth without gagging or feeling like they are going to throw up. Now is not the time to neglect brushing. Even if you weren't prone to gum disease before pregnancy, you might now notice swollen or tender gums that bleed when you brush. This is due to changing hormones and increased blood flow throughout your body. This provides a perfect environment for the bacteria living at the gum line, so brushing is even more important now that you are pregnant.

If the toothpaste bothers you, try different brands or flavors until you find one that you can tolerate. If the frothing toothpaste is the issue, spit it out more often. And although rinsing your mouth regularly does not take the place of good brushing, it is better than nothing. Do whatever you need to do to keep your teeth clean and healthy.

If vomiting is an issue, protect your teeth. Never brush immediately after the mouth is exposed to stomach acid. Once the outer layer of your teeth is softened by acid, the brushing action can remove the enamel. Rinsing with a solution of water and baking soda will neutralize the acid and allow the saliva to remineralize the tooth. If baking soda is not available, use liquid antacids or plain water. Some women have found that eating cheese can help protect the teeth from damage by neutralizing acids in the mouth as well as supplying additional calcium. If your teeth are exposed to acid repeatedly, such as daily, tell your dentist. To prevent dental erosion, your dentist may prescribe a fluoride rinse or gel.

I am always snacking. Is this bad for my teeth?

Many pregnant women who feel nauseated or have hypoglycemia eat frequent between-meal snacks—usually carbohydrates like crackers, bread, and cookies—to settle their stomachs. Foods high in starches promote tooth decay by increasing plaque, the invisible, sticky layer of harmful bacteria that constantly forms on teeth. The bacteria convert sugar and starch that remain in the mouth into acid that erodes tooth enamel. The longer sugars stay in the mouth, the longer and more dangerously the acids attack. After repeated attacks, tooth decay can result.

What's a hungry mom-to-be to do? Forgo some of the carbs, follow a well-balanced diet, and choose foods that are nutritious for you and your baby, such as raw fruits and vegetables and dairy products. And frequently brush or rinse your teeth.

How does my oral health change in pregnancy?

If you did not have your teeth cleaned before you found out you were pregnant, having your teeth cleaned by a dental hygienist or dentist early in your pregnancy may help prevent most problems. Hormone changes, mainly estrogen and progesterone, can cause many changes in the mouth. The same hormones that can make your ligaments looser in other joints during pregnancy can also cause looser teeth. If your teeth move around too easily, however, you may have severe periodontal disease and should be evaluated by a dentist as soon as possible.

Hormonal changes can also cause changes in saliva flow, either increasing or decreasing it. One of the body's primary defenses against tooth decay is saliva. It contains proteins and electrolytes that buffer and neutralize bacterial acids as well as minerals, like calcium and phosphorus, that help harden (or remineralize) teeth. During pregnancy, saliva composition may decrease in its buffering ability and mineral levels, increasing levels of bacteria. These bacteria can cause tooth decay or gum disease.

In other words, too little saliva (causing dry mouth, or xerostomia) or too much (pryalism) can increase the risk of tooth decay, so maintaining good oral hygiene habits is particularly important in pregnancy.

Your Baby's Teeth

How does what I eat in pregnancy affect my growing baby's teeth?

Good nutrition during pregnancy helps develop healthy teeth in the baby. Expectant moms should have adequate amounts of calcium, phosphorus, vitamin C, and vitamin D in their diets. When the fetus is between 14 weeks and 4 months, deficiencies in calcium, vitamin D, vitamin A, protein, and calories could result in oral defects.

- *Calcium.* You need 1,000 milligrams of calcium every day to build your baby's teeth and bones. Good calcium sources include fortified cereals, breads, oatmeal, and orange juice as well as collard greens.
- *Vitamin C.* Make sure you get at least 80 milligrams of vitamin C a day to help your body absorb iron. This mineral is essential to the formation of hemoglobin, which carries oxygen in the blood and is necessary for healthy cell growth and development. Broccoli, citrus fruits and juices, mangoes, and tomatoes are all good sources of vitamin C.
- *Vitamin D.* You need about 200 international units (IU) of vitamin D a day, primarily because you can't absorb calcium without it. Make sure the milk you buy is vitamin D–enriched, and try to get 15 minutes or so of sun

exposure every day. Other vitamin D sources include cod liver oil, egg yolks, and fatty cold-water fish such as wild Pacific salmon, sardines, and herring.

What happens with my baby's teeth during my pregnancy?

Your baby's teeth are developing, even though they don't show up on ultrasound, or even in that first toothless smile. There are three main stages in tooth development:

1. The first stage begins in the fetus at about 6 weeks of development. This is when the basic substance of the tooth forms.
2. Next, the hard tissue that surrounds the teeth is formed, at around 3 to 4 months of gestation.
3. After the child is born, the next stage occurs, when the tooth actually protrudes through the gum.

By the time babies are born, they have twenty primary teeth under the gum line and another sixteen permanent teeth ready and waiting.

Taking care of your teeth now will help you stay healthy and will help give your baby the best possible start too.

CHAPTER 7 ▼

Infants and Toddlers (Newborn to Age 4)

DuWain had perfected the act of ninja walking on tiptoe from the rocking chair to the crib. Once his wife finished nursing their 3-month-old daughter, Clara, to sleep, he'd do a stealth pickup and drop-off before Clara could wake up and demand more of their company. With a full belly and a satisfied smile on her face, Clara didn't make a sound as her dad tucked her in to sleep. Another crisis averted.

Between the feedings, diaper changes, and late-night cries, looking after the physical and emotional needs of a demanding baby can be exhausting. Once that baby becomes mobile, keeping him safe feels like a full-time job. Who has time to worry about baby teeth—especially since teeth don't even show up for months? But those baby teeth are important even before they appear, and even simple acts like wiping your baby's gums is the perfect start.

Milestones

A lot happens in your baby's mouth that first year. By baby's first birthday, the bottom and top front teeth will have come through the gums, and by the time your child is 3, all twenty baby teeth will be present and accounted for. With the baby teeth hard at work, the permanent incisors, canines, and molars will be starting to develop, with the crowns already complete.

When should my baby go to the dentist?

The American Academy of Pediatric Dentistry recommends a first dental visit shortly after the first tooth erupts and no later than a child's first birthday. Think of it as a well-child checkup for the teeth. This first visit is a good way to get to know the dentist and staff and to familiarize yourself with the office policies and procedures. The dentist will assess your child's dental development, establish correct fluoride levels, identify risk factors for decay, provide instructions on caring for your baby's mouth, and discuss ways to prevent oral and facial accidents and trauma as well as the relationship between diet and oral health. Check with your dental insurance policy to see if there are specific limitations on first visits.

An early visit is a good opportunity to establish a bond between the dentist and your child, setting the groundwork for a lifetime of good oral health. The sooner children become acquainted with the dentist, the better they will feel about the dental experience. Establish a dental home for your baby so that you have a resource if problems come up between annual visits. By the age of 3, your child will be well prepared for a complete oral examination, x-rays, a cleaning, and fluoride treatment.

Caring for Your Baby's Teeth

Before your baby's teeth erupt, get in the habit of washing the gums and tongue with a wet washcloth after feedings and during bath time. You don't need to use any toothpaste yet; just wrap the cloth or gauze around your index finger and rub it gently over the gums. Although bacteria in the mouth usually can't harm the gums before the teeth emerge, it can be difficult to tell when the teeth begin to push through, so start your baby's oral health care early. Plus, getting your baby used to having his mouth cleaned as part of his daily routine makes it easier to transition into tooth brushing later on.

When the first tooth erupts, begin brushing with a soft-bristled, small-head brush. The most important time to brush is at night, after the last feeding. By a year, your baby's teeth should be brushed at least twice a day (morning and night). You need only a smear of toothpaste for children younger than 2 years and a pea-sized amount for children ages 2 to 5. Begin flossing your child's teeth as soon as the surfaces of the teeth touch one another. Flossing should be done once a day, preferably with the evening brushing.

Make cleaning teeth fun by announcing, "We're going to get the sugar bugs off!" Count teeth in a silly way or sing a song about brushing to a fun tune. Try "Brush, brush, brush your teeth, up and down the gums" to the tune of "Row, Row, Row Your Boat." Or try this silly song, "Are Your Teeth Clean and White?" sung to the tune of "Do Your Ears Hang Low?" (You can find all the words to the song on many Internet sites.)

Are your teeth clean and white?
Do you brush them every night?
Do you brush them in the morning?
Do you brush them at night? (and so on)

Do I need to worry about fluoride for my baby?

Fluoride makes tooth enamel more resistant to demineralization (or thinning) by acids in the mouth and therefore helps prevent tooth decay. Pediatricians, dentists, and families should consider the child's risk of cavities, risk of dental fluorosis (a condition caused by ingesting too much fluoride), and the benefits of fluoride when deciding to use it in children younger than 2 years. If your water district doesn't add fluoride to the water supply, consult with your child's dentist or health care provider about the need for additional fluoride after your baby is 6 months old or the first tooth erupts. The main benefit of fluoride occurs after eruption, not before.

Fluoride can be applied topically, in fluoridated toothpaste, but only if your child is fully capable of spitting out the toothpaste and not at risk for swallowing it. Otherwise, it can be ingested systemically, in fluoride drops, which at one part per million are a safe and effective way to dramatically reduce dental decay, along with the cost of future dental treatment.

TABLE 7.1. When Do the Baby Teeth Come In and Fall Out?

	Age when they appear	Age when they fall out
Lower front four baby teeth	6-9 months	6-7 years
Upper front four baby teeth	7-10 months	7-8 years
First primary molars, right behind canines	13-19 months	10-12 years
Canine baby teeth, upper and lower	16-22 months	10-12 years
Second primary molars	about 2 years	10-12 years

Teething

When will my baby's teeth come in?

Although every child is different, most primary teeth (baby teeth) come in between the ages of 4 and 12 months. They usually begin to erupt around 6 months of age, and the eruption is completed by 24 to 36 months. Girls usually start teething slightly earlier than boys, and delays in tooth eruption can run in families.

Eruption is usually symmetrical (lower teeth before upper) in the following pattern for primary teeth: central incisors, lateral incisors, first molars, canines, second molars. A helpful way to remember the timing of primary eruption is the 7 + 4 rule. At 7 months of age, children often have their first teeth; at 11 months (4 months later), they usually have four teeth. At 15 months (4 months later), they have eight teeth, and so on. This pattern continues as follows:

19 months = 12 teeth
23 months = 16 teeth
27 months = 20 teeth

What if my baby's teeth are delayed?

A child's tooth timetable is thought to be hereditary, so if you want to guess when your child's teeth will start coming in, ask your parents when your teeth made their appearance. Primary teeth may not appear until later, with complete dentition (that is, all teeth in) delayed until age 4 or 5 for some children. Primary teeth are then retained in some children until they are 14 or 15.

> **Milk and Stomach Teeth**
>
> Your grandparents may refer to your child's first set of teeth as milk teeth, although this is no longer a common expression. Baby, or primary, teeth are also sometimes called deciduous, reborner, or temporary teeth. You may also have heard the bottom canines referred to as the stomach teeth and the top canines referred to as the eyeteeth.

Children with a growth hormone deficiency or Down syndrome may have delayed tooth eruption as well as an abnormal sequence of eruption. Some research suggests that delayed baby tooth eruption is associated with a 35 percent increased risk of requiring orthodontic treatment by the age of 30 years. If you're concerned, a visit to your child's dentist can reassure you that your baby's teeth are present in her jaw and will emerge in their own time.

Why are some babies born with teeth? Is it a problem?

In some rare cases (about one in every 3,000 births), babies are born with teeth already formed, called natal teeth. They might be "preteeth" that precede the arrival of the baby's real primary teeth, but they are usually just early baby teeth. You don't usually need to worry about them—nine times out of ten, they are lower incisors. As long as they don't cut into baby's tongue or mom's nipple while nursing, you don't have to do anything. If sharp edges become a problem, your child's dentist can file them down to decrease the risk of injury.

If they are supernumerary, or extra teeth, they are improperly formed and are often loose. Because of the danger of being aspirated (inhaled), early teeth may need to be extracted. Sometimes an x-ray will be recommended to see if the teeth are extra or just early risers. If an early tooth needs to be extracted, remember there will be a gap until the secondary teeth appear later in elementary school.

How can I tell when my baby is teething?

Teething can cause discomfort for your baby, as well as many sleepless nights for you. New parents are often confused about what signs to look for when baby is developing new teeth. During teething periods, your baby may exhibit increased biting, drooling, gum rubbing, sucking, irritability, wakefulness, ear rubbing, facial rash, decreased appetite for solid foods, and mild fever. The symptoms of teething are now known to be extremely mild. But because babies, at around 6 months old, start to lose the immunity passed on by their mothers, they coincidentally tend to pick up a lot of new infections around the time that teething begins. A fever higher than 101 degrees Fahrenheit is not associated with teething and warrants a call to your child's health care provider.

Teething's Bad Reputation

Teething has received a lot of bad press over the years. During the nineteenth century, babies' gums were cut to assist with teething, and as recently as the 1930s, teething was still thought to cause death. Symptoms like vomiting, bronchitis, loose stools, and fever are often blamed on teething, but they are not associated with it. One study found that of every fifty babies seen by a physician for symptoms caregivers related to teething, forty-eight were found to have an illness not teething related. If you think your baby is ill, check with your health care provider.

What can I do about teething pain and discomfort?

Unfortunately, new teeth coming in can be uncomfortable for babies and caregivers. Lightly rubbing your baby's gums with gauze pads several times a day will remove the thin layer of plaque that forms on their gums, thus lessening the pain as the teeth come in. This massaging and close contact is soothing for most babies. Your baby may enjoy sucking on the gauze or your finger.

Refrigerated teething rings, biscuits, pacifiers, spoons, clean wet washcloths, and frozen bagels or bananas are all good choices for cranky babies to chew on. The coolness acts as an anesthetic for the gums. Note that teething rings should be placed in the refrigerator only, not the freezer, to prevent tissue damage.

Topically applied teething gels or ointments will temporarily numb your baby's gums and reduce discomfort, but read the label carefully: adult products should not be used on children. You can also use a barrier cream on your baby's chin to help prevent soreness from continual drooling.

Why do my child's baby teeth look so big?

Sometimes baby teeth do look a little out of place on cute baby faces. It's all about perspective! Those baby teeth may seem to loom large in your little one's face now, but they will stay the same size while your child's head keeps growing over the next few years. It may take a while, but those teeth will look just right on your precious pre-schooler's face.

There may also be gaps between your baby's teeth that look worrisome. But gaps between baby teeth may mean your child will have enough room for permanent teeth without crowding. Maybe you can avoid orthodontist visits! Most of these spaces close as the permanent teeth reach their final positions.

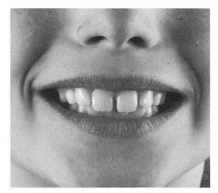

Normal gaps between primary teeth.
© Can Stock Photo Inc./jc_cards

Feedings and Healthy Teeth

How does breastfeeding affect my baby's teeth?

Breastfeeding is best for baby for many reasons, including ideal nutritional content, better absorption, fewer food-related allergies, better immunologic defenses, and, of course, it saves money. Breastfeeding also promotes the proper development of an infant's oral cavity, including improved shaping of the hard palate (the roof of the mouth). It encourages proper alignment of teeth and fewer problems with malocclusion (improper bite). Breastfeeding infants also have a lower risk for tooth decay than nonbreastfed babies. Milk proteins in breast milk protect the enamel on the teeth, and the antibacterial qualities in breast milk stop the bacteria from using the lactose in breast milk in the same way as regular sugar.

Some myths persist regarding breastfeeding women's teeth, particularly one about nursing moms getting the calcium leached out of their teeth. Breastfeeding will not harm your teeth, but breastfeeding moms do need adequate calcium intake—from foods like milk, cheese, and fortified cereals and juice. The recommended calcium intake for women ages 19 to 50, whether or not they are breastfeeding, is 1,000 milligrams a day. Calcium helps prevent bone density loss and will help your teeth stay healthy and strong.

How does bottle feeding affect teeth?

Infant formula typically contains more sugar than breast milk does. Bacteria that cause tooth decay love sugar. In fact, the only three ingredients bacteria need to thrive are sugar, warmth, and water. Bottle feeding offers all of these, especially if bottles are left in an infant's crib all night. The best defense is good oral hygiene, which is an important part of every baby's care, regardless of the type of feeding offered. The gums should be gently cleaned with water and a soft cloth or gauze pad as part of bath time and after feedings.

Mom's Dental Care while Nursing

As you know, any medications you take while you're nursing get passed along to your baby. If you need to have dental work done, talk to your dentist and your child's pediatrician about any medications that may be used and how to minimize your baby's exposure. For some heavy-duty sedation medications, you may want to pump and dump for a few feedings afterward. Local anesthetics such as lidocaine and bupivacaine are most commonly used, and breastfeeding should be withheld as a precaution for at least 4 hours after the use of these drugs.

Are some bottle and pacifier nipples better than others?

The type of nipple used on a bottle or pacifier may have an effect on the growth of the jaw and the development of muscles and swallowing patterns. Bottles and pacifiers come in a variety of nipple shapes, including:

- Orthodontic: a flattened nipple that looks and feels most like a breast
- Angled: a slanted nipple that automatically tilts into baby's mouth
- Vented: a nipple with a tiny hole to let air into the bottle while your baby sucks, minimizing gas

Try various shapes and let your baby's mouth decide. Talk to your child's dentist and pediatrician about recommended options.

What is "baby bottle mouth"?

Many parents give their babies a bottle in bed to help them fall asleep. Most people fill the bottle with milk, formula, fruit juice, or water mixed with a sweetening agent, such as Karo syrup. Unfortunately, as the baby falls asleep, his tongue and the nipple on the bottle pool the liquid around certain teeth. The acidic, sugary content of these liquids can cause severe tooth decay. This is called nursing bottle or baby bottle mouth.

Imagine this: you have a bottle of natural fruit juice that you sip throughout the day, taking a sip, putting it down, then picking it up for another sip

---

Feeding Tips to Prevent Tooth Decay

- Do not fill your child's bottle with fluids that are high in sugar, such as juice, sports drinks, or soft drinks.
- Give children ages 6 to 12 months only formula or breast milk to drink in bottles.
- Put your child to bed with a bottle of water only—not juice, milk, or other drinks.
- Remove the bottle or stop nursing when your child has fallen asleep.
- Avoid letting your child walk around using a bottle or sippy cup of juice or milk as a pacifier.
- Avoid prolonged use of pacifiers.

- Never dip the pacifier in honey, sugar, or syrup. Honey should never be given to infants under 1 year of age, due to the risk of botulism spores.
- Begin to teach your child to drink from a cup at around 6 months of age. Try to stop using a bottle by the time your child is 12 to 14 months.
- Check your child's mouth often, looking for any unusual red or swollen areas or any dark spots on your child's teeth. If you see anything unusual, make a dentist appointment within the next few weeks.

20 minutes later. Each sip allows the sugar to coat your teeth. The bacteria in your mouth metabolize the sugar, turning it into acid. This acid remains active for about 20 minutes, at which time you take another sip, starting the whole sugar/acid cycle over again. One bottle may last a whole day, but that bottle contains enough sugar to cause major damage to your teeth.

Baby bottle mouth, or early childhood cavities, usually occurs in the upper front teeth but can affect any tooth. Some children experience decay so severe that the teeth cannot be repaired and need to be removed, which is painful, traumatic, and costly.

How much juice should my baby have each day?

For babies and toddlers, minimize juice consumption and allow juice drinking only from a cup (not a bottle or sippy cup). The American Academy of Pediatrics recommends the following guidelines:

- Do not give juice to children younger than 1 year of age.
- Give fruit juice only with meals.
- Limit fruit juice to 4 to 6 oz/day for children 1 to 6 years of age.
- Limit juice to 8 to 12 oz/day for children 7 to 18 years of age.

Nutrition for a Healthy Mouth

Feeding very young children can be a challenge. Whether your child is a picky eater or always hungry, the food choices you make can play an important role in his oral health. Constant eating, or grazing, is hard on teeth, so plan your child's foods for the day with three meals and two snacks. Offering choices is important for children anxious to be independent, but limit the options of foods high in sugar, such as cake, cookies, or candy, and offer them only at mealtimes. Avoid foods that stick to the surface of the teeth and are difficult to remove. Examples of sticky foods include Fruit Roll-Ups, gummies, dried fruit (raisins), and certain candies, like caramel. Choose fresh fruits, vegetables, and whole grain snacks. Limit juices and avoid carbonated beverages altogether. Soda should be considered an infrequent treat throughout a lifetime, even for teenagers and adults.

My baby won't fall asleep without a bottle. What can I do?

The best bet is to stop night feedings once the teeth erupt. Most children are physically able to tolerate a prolonged fast around 6 months of age, which is when the teeth typically begin to come through. To calm a crying baby, try to use methods other than feeding, such as giving him a small blanket, favorite toy, or stuffed animal, or just rocking or singing to him.

If you must give your baby a bottle in bed, be sure to fill it with only water. Never put baby to bed with a bottle of formula, breast milk, regular milk, juice, or soda. If you elect to feed on demand at night, wipe your baby's teeth clean after feedings. Introduce a cup as soon as your child can sit unsupported (usually around 6 months of age), and try to eliminate the bottle completely by 1 year of age. Remember to never prop a bottle up for your baby and always remove it right away once your baby is done feeding.

Pacifiers and Thumb Sucking

Is it okay for my baby to sleep with a pacifier instead of a bottle?

Research indicates that pacifier use may actually decrease the risk of sudden infant death syndrome (SIDS), so go ahead and offer a pacifier at naptime and bedtime. Pacifier use throughout the first year of life is generally appropriate within these guidelines suggested by the American Academy of Pediatrics Task Force on Sudden Infant Death Syndrome:

- Offer the pacifier when placing your baby down for sleep but do not reinsert it after she falls asleep. If your baby refuses the pacifier, don't force her to take it.
- Never coat pacifiers in any sweet solution.
- Clean pacifiers often and replace them regularly.
- If you are breastfeeding your baby, wait a month before introducing the pacifier to ensure that breastfeeding is firmly established.
- Never use a pacifier to replace or delay meals. Offer it when you are certain your child is not hungry.

- Pacifiers should have ventilation holes and a shield wider than your child's mouth (at least 1¼ inches in diameter).
- Pacifiers should be one piece and made of a durable material, replaced when worn, and never tied by a string to the crib or around your child's neck or hand.
- Physiologic pacifiers are preferable to conventional pacifiers because they may have fewer dental effects.

Also, if the pacifier falls on the floor, don't pop it in your own mouth to "clean" it, because this will introduce your own oral bacteria.

When should my child stop using a pacifier?

Dental effects from pacifier use are generally reversible and unlikely to cause any long-term problems if a child stops using the pacifier by age 3. It is important to break the habit before the permanent teeth erupt and well before baby teeth start getting loose, preferably beginning by age 2. Long-term sucking can cause problems with permanent teeth that can only be corrected with braces:

- The top front teeth slant out (overbite or open bite).
- The bottom front teeth tilt in.
- The upper and lower jaws are misaligned.
- The roof of the mouth is narrower side-to-side (crossbite).

After your child is 1 year old, limit the pacifier to naps and bedtime so that it doesn't interfere with speech. Sucking on a pacifier locks a child's mouth in an unnatural position, making it more difficult for him to develop his tongue and lip muscles normally. Frequent pacifier use can cause the tongue to push forward between the teeth, setting the stage for the development of a lisp when producing the *s* and *z* sounds. Pacifiers should be the newborn size, even as your baby ages, to decrease the likelihood of dental and speech problems.

Will thumb sucking cause problems with my son's teeth?

Thumb sucking is another form of non-nutritive sucking that isn't a problem with infants, but it can be a hard habit to break as they get older. Thumb suckers usually continue the habit longer than pacifier users, in part because pacifiers can eventually be taken away, but thumbs can't. Long-term thumb sucking can lead to various problems. It might interfere with the development of your child's permanent teeth by changing the shape and size of his palate, so he may need a retainer or braces that he may not have needed otherwise. Thumb suckers can also develop teeth that stick out, a bite that doesn't close properly, or possibly a tongue thrust, which might result in a lisp.

How can I help my daughter stop sucking her thumb?

If your child is still sucking her thumb by age 2, it may be time to start discouraging the behavior. The American Dental Association offers these tips:

- Praise children for not sucking, instead of scolding them when they are.
- Children often suck their thumbs when feeling insecure or needing comfort. Focus on correcting the cause of the anxiety and comforting your child.
- For an older child, involve her in choosing the method of stopping.
- Your child's dentist can offer encouragement to your child and explain what could happen to her teeth if she does not stop sucking.
- If the above tips don't work, remind your child of the habit by bandaging her thumb or putting a sock on her hand at night. Your child's dentist or pediatrician might prescribe a bitter medication to coat the thumb or the use of a mouth appliance.

Other Dental Concerns in Infants and Toddlers

What are the little bumps on the top of my baby's mouth?

Found in 80 percent of newborns, Epstein's pearls are whitish yellow protein-filled cysts that form on the palate, or roof of the mouth. Also called gingival cysts of the newborn, they usually disappear within two weeks. Bohn's nodules are similar but are located on the gums. Both conditions are harmless, although they sometimes worry new parents.

What is thrush?

If your baby needs antibiotics, or if you take them while breastfeeding, he might develop a case of thrush, a common and harmless yeast infection. Antibiotics kill off good bacteria that keep yeast in check, sometimes resulting in what looks like cottage cheese or milk curds on the sides, roof, and sometimes tongue of a baby's mouth. Thrush happens most often in babies 2 months old or younger, but it can appear in older babies, too.

If you see white spots in your baby's mouth, gently touch them with a fingertip wrapped in clean gauze. Thrush won't come off easily, and if it does, you'll see a raw, red area underneath, which may bleed. The infection should go away on its own within a few weeks, but you can call your pediatrician for an oral fungal medication called nystatin. Using an applicator or a finger, you'll paint the medicine on the white patches several times a day for ten days.

If you're breastfeeding, the yeast infection can affect your nipple, which can be painful. Plus, you and your baby can pass the infection back and forth. You don't have to stop breastfeeding, but you may want to talk to a lactation consultant or your child's pediatrician about the best way to treat it.

Do premature babies have particular dental problems?

Some prematurely born babies will develop stained teeth and enamel hypoplasia, which causes white spots on teeth. Others may have more serious problems. Tooth discoloration generally occurs only in premature infants with high bilirubin levels. A yellow or brown color, which appears only on the primary teeth, cannot be removed by brushing or a dental office cleaning.

Another common problem, called palatal groove, occurs in premature babies who have to be intubated in the neonatal intensive care unit

(NICU). The tube causes a narrow groove in the roof of the mouth, also called the hard palate. The longer the intubation time, the more likely a palatal groove will develop, although it can form in as little as a week. Some hospitals provide a protective device called a palate plate or palatal stabilizing device to protect the baby's palate during intubation. The tube can be retaped every 24 hours and moved side-to-side to avoid the groove.

Overall, studies have shown that the groove disappears with time. Although a palatal groove can lead to teeth crowding, poor positioning of teeth, sucking or speech problems, or hearing difficulties, there are usually no irreversible side effects on teeth from early intubation.

Some children born prematurely will require a palate expander or other dental appliance to correct any problems. A pediatric dentist with experience in this area can respond best to any concerns you have.

Baby Steps

Caregivers play a critical role in creating a healthy start for babies. From the beginning, you can do a lot to keep your baby's gums and new teeth healthy and bright.

CHAPTER 8

Early Childhood (Ages 5 to 8)

"Look, Mommy!" Jackson shouted from the monkey bars, where he and his friend Noah were playing while their mothers watched from a nearby bench. Jackson ran toward them, pointing to one of his bottom middle teeth. "It's loose!" he squealed with delight, wiggling it around with his tongue.

Getting a closer look, his mother replied, "Yes, it is! I'd better let the tooth fairy know about this. She'll want to plan a special trip." Turning to Noah's mother, she said, "Jackson just turned 5 last week. Isn't it a little early for him to be losing teeth? His older brother didn't lose a tooth until he was almost 7."

"I don't think he's too young," Noah's mother replied. Although Noah hadn't lost a tooth yet at 6½, nothing about Jackson's loose tooth seemed out of the ordinary.

Jackson's mom wanted to make sure he hadn't knocked the tooth loose at school earlier in the day. "Did you hurt yourself today?" she asked. "Did you bump your mouth while you were playing?" Jackson shook his head no and grinned widely to show off his wiggly tooth.

When Jackson's mom called the dentist, he assured her that it sounded like Jackson's loose tooth was just a normal part of growing up. Some children lose teeth earlier than others. He told her there wasn't anything to do but wait for the tooth to continue to work its way loose. Eventually it would come out easily.

Milestones

Ages 5 to 8 are exciting times, from that memorable first lost tooth, usually in the front, to the silly smiles that come with it. As your child's permanent incisors make their debut, his permanent molars are developing behind the scenes. You may notice that your little one loses his baby face appearance around this time, as the growth in the upper part of his face is almost done.

These years are also crucial in laying the foundation for a healthy smile. What happens during this phase heavily influences your child's lifelong dental health.

What to Expect at the Dentist

At this age, children should already be familiar with the dentist's office and comfortable with routine procedures like the examination and cleaning. The American Academy of Pediatric Dentistry also recommends fluoride treatments for children at each six-month checkup and x-rays at least once a year. Your child's diet and ability to brush and floss effectively can affect how often x-rays are needed.

Despite our best efforts to make children feel safe and comfortable at the dentist, some children still suffer from intense anxiety. If you and your child's dentist are unable to calm these fears, the dentist may use nitrous oxide to make the visit more productive and more comfortable for your child. Nitrous oxide (also called laughing gas) is commonly used to relax children and to create a more positive experience with the dentist. Not every child is alike, however, and dental staff may recommend other ways to reduce stress and anxiety according to your child's specific needs. Collaborate with the dentist to find a solution for any dental anxiety your child is experiencing since dental checkups need to happen regularly.

Caring for Your Child's Teeth

Between the ages of 5 and 8, your child should start to show an interest in brushing her own teeth. This is important, because it will help her develop good habits, but children at this age still need close supervision and help in brushing. Children should brush at least twice daily, once in the morning and once before bedtime. To make sure that all teeth are being brushed, work with your child to develop a tooth-brushing sequence that covers all teeth (see chapter 2). Most of the time should be spent on the back chewing surfaces, where cavities usually develop first.

It always seems like a fight to get my daughter to brush. What can I do?

Children at this age are beginning to exert their independence and want to be in control. Brushing teeth is no different. Although getting children to brush their teeth isn't always easy, the teeth must be brushed. Here are a few tips to encourage a lifetime of good dental health.

1. Let your child pick out her supplies, including toothbrushes, toothpastes, and floss. Take your child to the store to pick out her favorite characters or colors. She will be more interested in brushing if she is involved from the beginning.

2. Try a power-operated toothbrush. A child may find it more fun than a regular toothbrush. Today, there are many options for power toothbrushes, including kid-friendly, inexpensive disposable ones that you throw out after a few months, once the battery power is gone.

3. Set a timer. A simple egg timer or a cool digital timer will work. Set it for 2 minutes and have your child brush until it goes off. By the way, this is about the same amount of time it takes to sing "Happy Birthday to You" three times, another trick that works for some parents, especially if you don't have a timer handy.

4. Brush as a family so your child can mimic good tooth-brushing and flossing habits. If your child sees you doing it, she will want to join too.

5. Maintain a schedule. Children like to know exactly what to expect and when to expect it. If you stick to a routine with regular tooth-brushing times, it will become a part of your child's day, minimizing the chance for complaining or conflicts.

Why is our dentist recommending sealants?

Many dentists begin to recommend sealants for children when per-manent teeth start to grow in. Sealants consist of a thin coating applied to teeth to help keep them cavity-free. Even if your child brushes and flosses every day, it is difficult (sometimes impossible) to clean all the tiny grooves and pits on certain teeth. Food and bacteria build up in these crevices, making them a perfect environment for tooth decay. Although varying views about sealants exist, much scientific evidence suggests that they are an effective preventive therapy to protect a child's permanent teeth. This is particularly important for the molars, in the back of the mouth, where effective brushing is usually more difficult. In general, seal-ants provide an extra layer that "seals out" food and plaque, keeping them from reaching the surface of the tooth, which reduces the risk of decay. (For more information about dental sealants, see chapter 4.)

When should my child begin flossing?

Flossing removes particles and plaque between the teeth that regular brushing misses. You should begin to floss your child's teeth regularly by age 4. At around age 8, most children can start flossing themselves. How-ever, if your child has problems with flossing, feel free to continue doing it yourself until he is ready.

For some children, flossing is easier with a floss holder (or flosser), a short piece of floss held by a small plastic "y." Floss holders are espe-cially helpful for youngsters who have not yet fully developed their fine motor skills. To use one, your child places the floss at the top of the holder between each tooth.

You can get one-time-use disposable floss holders at any local drug-store or supermarket. They even come in lots of fun colors and shapes, including dinosaurs and princesses. Alternatively, you can purchase a reusable holder, where your replace just the floss after each use.

My daughter's baby teeth are crooked.
Is it possible to straighten them?

Tooth-straightening appliances slowly move teeth into position. Although they may work on baby teeth, doing so is "off label," meaning the treating dentist would be acting alone and not in line with the manufacturer's recommendations. These appliances are supposed to be used only on permanent teeth, after all baby teeth are gone. Baby teeth are often crooked, ungainly, and sort of unattractive. Hang in there and wait for those permanent teeth to start coming in. If her permanent teeth are crooked, a visit to the orthodontist is in order once she is a little older.

Losing Baby Teeth

Most cultures view teething as a rite of passage—the nursing baby starts to eat solid foods when teeth come in; the infant becomes a young adult when all the baby teeth are lost and replaced by permanent teeth. Unless they hit their teeth in a fall or have other dental trauma, most children start losing their primary (or baby) teeth around age 6 or 7, give or take a year or two. It can start to happen as early as 4 or as late as 8. In general, girls usually lose teeth a bit earlier than boys.

Typically, baby teeth fall out in the order in which they came in. The bottom two front teeth are usually the first to go, followed by the front top two. It generally takes a few months from the time a tooth becomes loose until it falls out. A baby tooth does not usually become loose until the permanent tooth below pushes it up to take its place.

During early childhood, the permanent tooth begins to grow just under the baby tooth. The root of the baby tooth starts to dissolve, and the tooth becomes loose. It can take as long as three and half years for the baby tooth to lose its roots and be replaced by the permanent tooth. The crown of the permanent tooth is the first part to develop and grow into the space left by the root of the baby tooth. When the crown erupts, it is covered by a cuticle, a film that protects the enamel and is slowly worn away by chewing and tooth brushing.

TABLE 8.1. When Do the Permanent Teeth Come In?

Tooth order	Tooth name	Age when tooth erupts	Age when root is fully formed
1	Central incisor	7 to 8 years	10 to 11 years
2	Lateral incisor	8 to 9 years	11 to 12 years
3	Canine	9 to 12 years	14 to 15 years
4	First premolar (bicuspid)	10 to 11 years	13 to 14 years
5	Second premolar (bicuspid)	11 to 12 years	13 to 15 years
6	First molar	6 to 7 years	8 to 10 years
7	Second molar	12 to 13 years	15 to 16 years
8	Third molar	17 to 21 years	19 to 23 years

Children normally have twenty baby teeth, and by age 12 or 13, they have usually lost all twenty, which are replaced by twenty-eight permanent teeth. The final four teeth—the wisdom teeth, or third molars—do not appear until the late teens or early twenties.

What does it mean for a tooth to "erupt"?

Teeth are formed in the jawbone and must grow through the bone and the gum covering into the mouth. This process is call eruption. When a baby tooth falls out, the adult tooth is usually right underneath the gums, ready to erupt.

The final position of a tooth is determined by an interplay of the tongue, lips, and cheeks. The tongue exerts outward pressure on the teeth while the lips and cheeks provide a balancing inward force. Thumb sucking and tongue thrusting can also provide pressure and force teeth out of position.

My daughter lost her first tooth well before kindergarten. Is this going to cause any problems?

Some children lose a baby tooth early, before the permanent tooth is ready to erupt. Most often this is due to an accident or dental disease.

Whatever the cause, be sure to consult your child's dentist, especially if your child loses her first tooth before age 4. Sometimes the dentist will decide to put in a space maintainer, a custom-fit metal placeholder that is inserted where a baby tooth fell out too soon. This space maintainer will prevent unwanted movement, or "drift," of baby teeth and permanent teeth until the adult tooth is ready to erupt. It maintains the ideal space for the developing permanent tooth, with the goal of limiting future orthodontic problems.

My son is 7 years old and still has not lost a tooth. Should I be concerned?

Not necessarily. Although most children begin losing their baby teeth around age 6, some children don't lose teeth until they are well into their seventh or even eighth year. Parents should not worry; this is perfectly normal. Most likely everything is fine, but x-rays may be recommended to make sure all the teeth are present under the gums. If your child started teething late, there is a good chance he will also lose teeth later than classmates and friends. Losing teeth late may also be hereditary. If either parent lost baby teeth late, your child might lose them at an older age too.

If permanent teeth start coming in before your child's baby teeth fall out, your child's dentist may opt to pull the baby teeth to make room. Extracting baby teeth is often necessary if the baby teeth remain tight, especially if this causes the adult teeth to erupt slowly into a double row. Ideally, there is lots of space between all the baby teeth.

How can I make it easier for my child to eat with loose teeth?

Young children with loose teeth often say that it's hard to eat. To make it easier for your child, you may want to chop or mince meats and cook fruits and vegetables thoroughly. Test cooked foods by piercing them with the tip of a sharp knife or a fork. If the knife or fork goes in easily, the food is ready. Experiment to see whether the food can be eaten as is once it is cooked or if it needs to be mashed. Some foods, such as avocados and bananas, can be mashed raw, while others need to be cooked completely first. Mashing is easiest to do on a flat surface, such as a plate, or in a large bowl. Mash foods with the back of a fork or with a spoon.

Avoid giving chewy or hard foods to your child when her teeth are loose, because these foods sometimes cause discomfort. Chewy candy, gum, and hard foods may also cause the tooth to fall out prematurely, causing pain and possibly excessive bleeding.

Is it safe to pull a loose tooth?

Although parents have been pulling teeth for generations, forcing your child's baby tooth out too soon can be painful and possibly lead to infection and excessive bleeding. The best choice is to have your child wiggle it loose using his tongue or finger. Eventually the tooth will seem to come out on its own with minimal bleeding or discomfort. If there is no root left, it should come out easily. Don't ever force it, and never tie a string to it. If this root is only partially dissolved, it could break and become infected. Very rarely, a loose tooth that refuses to come out will need to be pulled by a dentist.

How do I stop the bleeding after a tooth falls out?

It is normal to have some bleeding after a baby tooth falls out. Have your child lean over a sink to spit out the blood and avoid swallowing it. To minimize the bleeding, use a clean, damp gauze pad to put consistent pressure on the gum until bleeding subsides. It should take no more than 20 to 30 minutes for the bleeding to stop. If the bleeding continues for more than half an hour, seek advice from a medical professional.

Generally, you do not need to do anything else, although the newly

> **Mouth Power!**
>
> What is the secret to a healthy smile? Taking good care of your teeth! Mouth Power, created by the National Museum of Dentistry in partnership with the American Dental Association, is an entertaining and educational Web site featuring the character Mouthie. In Mouthie's online laboratory, children can do fun activities that teach them about dental health, from taking care of their teeth to making healthy food choices. Available in English and Spanish at www.mouthpower.org.

exposed gum may be tender. Applying a small, refrigerated cold pack wrapped in gauze can help relieve minor pain and discomfort. Do not place an ice pack directly on the mouth or gums, however, because it may cause further irritation or injury.

My son's tooth fell out, and it has holes in it. What's wrong with it?

Baby teeth can decay quickly because the enamel is softer and thinner than that of adult teeth. Sometimes decay is present as the baby teeth come in. Sugary fluids like milk and juice can stick to the baby teeth and cause decay. If cavities are not addressed in baby teeth, they will continue to decay. Cavities can turn teeth black and create holes. Parents should always be attentive to any holes in baby teeth and tell their child's dentist at the next checkup.

Why does my 5-year-old grind her teeth at night?

When children grind their teeth, especially at night, it can be so loud that it worries many parents. Unlike adult teeth grinders, however, grinding at night is normal for young children. There are two main reasons they might do this. First, grinding places pressure on the roots of the baby teeth over the developing adult teeth, which stimulates the natural destruction of the roots of the baby teeth. This process is ultimately responsible for shedding the baby teeth when the adult teeth are ready to erupt. Grinding teeth also helps the adult teeth to erupt into their most stable positions within the mouth.

Nighttime teeth grinding (also called bruxism) in children usually does not require any treatment. Most children outgrow this. In fact, the

---

Tooth Dreams

Having dreams about losing your teeth? You might feel as though you're losing your youth. Having dreams about having your teeth pulled? You might be feeling pulled to go in a direction you don't want to go. Teeth are common symbols in dreams, and their dream meanings have been analyzed for thousands of years across different cultures. In Greek culture, dreaming about teeth or losing your teeth suggests that someone in your family will be sick, while the Chinese say that when your teeth fall out in your dreams, it means you're telling lies. Or your toothy dreams could just be your subconscious reminding you to schedule a checkup with your dentist.

grinding typically decreases around the ages of 6 to 8, and children tend to stop grinding altogether by age 12.

Tooth Fairy Lore

Teething rituals have been around since the dawn of time. Everything that belonged to a child, from hair and nail clippings to baby teeth, was revered and sometimes thought to need special protection from evil spirits. In customs around the world, dogs, rabbits, pigs, birds, and even rats are responsible for protecting children's baby teeth. Children's teeth may be planted, thrown onto the roof, tossed into fires, hidden in slippers, or even dipped in gold.

The current version of the tooth fairy didn't make an appearance until the early 1900s, as a generalized good fairy with mystical powers. Over time, she has morphed into a symbol of childlike fantasy and whimsy, no longer needed to protect children's teeth from being inhabited by the forces of evil. Today, a child loses a baby tooth and puts it under her pillow, and that night, the tooth fairy exchanges it for a small gift or money.

The tooth fairy grew slowly in popularity over the first half of the twentieth century. Around the 1950s, she began to appear in numerous children's books, cartoons, jokes, and so on along with a heightened focus on children's dental hygiene. Parents happily bought into the idea, and the tooth fairy became part of the family. The tooth fairy became commercialized in the 1980s when special pillows, dolls, decorative tooth containers, and banks could be found in stores.

Belief in the tooth fairy is generally short lived. Although children can lose their teeth until age 10 or 11, or even a bit older, most kids stop believing around age 7 or 8. Regardless, parents usually continue to play the tooth fairy, and children still look forward to their reward until all their baby teeth are gone.

While your child still believes, she might enjoy receiving personalized letters from the tooth fairy and have fun with the activities at www.ncohf .org (click on America's Tooth Fairy Kids Club).

What is the going rate for lost teeth?

The custom of leaving monetary gifts for lost teeth varies tremendously. Rosemary Wells is known as the world's leading tooth fairy authority and has studied the exchange rate for teeth from 1900 to 1980. In general, the tooth fairy kept up with inflation. The going rate had increased from about a dime in the mid-1960s to nearly two bucks in the 1990s. More recent data suggest that the average value received by children today is about $1 to $5 per tooth. However, it can still range between 25 cents to $20 or more, depending on the family.

Nonmonetary gifts, such as a sticker, small toy, or book, are becoming increasingly popular these days. Parents should decide on what the gift is to be before the event, so they're not caught unprepared at the last minute. The gift the tooth fairy leaves the first time generally sets a precedent for all future visits, although some families explain that the first tooth lost fetches a higher amount than any subsequent teeth. Shedding teeth can be annoying and frightening but is also a sign of growing up. Since many young children are scared of change, even losing a tooth, a treat for a lost tooth can help soften the experience and the uncertainty.

> **Lost Baby Teeth around the World**
>
> In Spain, a small mouse (called Ratoncito Perez) leaves a surprise under a little one's pillow when a child loses a tooth. In Kyrgyzstan, a child will hide his tooth in a piece of bread and give it to an animal with desirable teeth. A mouse will give the child healthy white sharp teeth, while a dog might give a child yellow stained teeth. Children in Cambodia toss their lower teeth on the roof and bury their upper teeth in the ground. They hope that the new teeth will grow toward the old teeth and be straight.

What if my child loses his lost tooth?

Many children believe that they must have their lost tooth to put under their pillow for the tooth fairy to visit. Unfortunately, young children often lose their lost teeth. Sometimes they swallow it, or it goes down the drain or falls out on the playground. If your child has a tooth extracted at the dentist's office, she may not be allowed to bring it home, depending on the office policy. If your child's lost or extracted tooth is not available, have her write a special note to the tooth fairy explaining the situation and leave the note under her pillow. As far as the tooth fairy is concerned, a note from a child is just as magical as the lost tooth.

The tooth fairy "forgot" to visit. What should I say?

Most children understand that even the tooth fairy makes mistakes or gets too busy to retrieve every tooth the first night it is left. Some families add a little bit extra as a "late payment" penalty. Overall, children are pretty flexible and are likely to believe whatever excuse you make for the tooth fairy's neglect.

What does the tooth fairy do with all those teeth?

There's no consensus. Some parents suggest that the tooth turns into the surprise left under the pillow, while others describe how the tooth fairy's minions collect teeth, neatly label them, and file them away in a museum-like castle inhabited by the tooth fairy and her helpers. Still others tell their children that she makes them into beautiful fairy jewelry or that the old baby teeth get recycled for new babies. One creative dad explained that the rattle you hear when you shake a can of spray paint is a kid's tooth that the tooth fairy sold to the paint company.

Your Child's Changing Face

In addition to the growing teeth, the bones of the face also grow during this period. The jawbone needs to grow to accommodate thirty-two permanent teeth in place of twenty baby teeth. In fact, the jaw grows at a faster rate than the rest of the face, eventually measuring up to one-third the size of the face. If the jaw does not grow sufficiently, crowding or impacted teeth may result. An orthodontist can help address these problems.

My daughter's new permanent teeth look too big for her smile. Is this normal?

Your child's new smile may be a little awkward for a while. The adult teeth are bigger than the baby teeth. Brand new permanent teeth usually have ridges on the biting edges at first (until they get worn down by chewing), and the teeth may be slightly less white than the baby teeth. As more adult teeth grow in, this color difference becomes less noticeable.

My son's baby teeth were nice and straight, but his permanent teeth are coming in crooked. Why is this?

Adult teeth can grow in crooked, overlapping, or twisted for various reasons. A history of thumb sucking, mouth breathing, tongue thrusting, pacifier use, or prolonged bottle use can significantly affect growing teeth. Crooked teeth often occur when children begin to lose their teeth earlier than average. Some children's mouths are still too small for their teeth. This causes crowding and may cause teeth to shift. Crooked teeth and jaw size can be inherited, too, so think back to your own tooth development for some insight into your child's dental future.

Sometimes, crooked teeth can be caused by an extra tooth that interferes with the normal path of eruption. Extra teeth sometimes need to be extracted to allow the normal eruption of the permanent teeth.

Why does my child have two rows of teeth right next to each other?

The process of losing baby teeth and growing adult teeth takes place over several years. As permanent teeth grow in, the roots of baby teeth usually dissolve, allowing them to fall out easily. This usually happens smoothly, with baby teeth falling out before the new ones start to grow in, but sometimes minor problems occur. One of the most common problems related to timing is a condition commonly called shark teeth, or ectopic eruption. This means that a permanent tooth is growing in before the baby tooth is lost. Since the baby tooth is in the way, the new tooth grows in behind it. The child then has two rows of teeth at once, similar to a shark's double row of teeth. This can occur with either the lower or the upper set of teeth. Although most common around age 6, "shark teeth" can appear any time from when a child starts losing teeth to when this process is completed, usually around age 11.

This condition usually resolves on its own. As the new tooth continues to grow in, the baby tooth will eventually become loose and fall out. If not, a dentist can extract the tooth. Once the baby tooth is gone, the new permanent tooth will typically move forward into the correct place over the next few weeks or months.

CHAPTER 9 ▼

Middle Childhood (Ages 9 to 12)

"It's Thursday—don't forget your sneakers for practice after school," yelled Ken's mom to her 11-year-old son as he raced around the house trying to avoid yet another tardy slip. "And please, please, please brush your teeth this morning. I checked your toothbrush last night and it was dry!" "Okay, Mom, okay. I'll do it." After a flurry of activity and one barely caught school bus, Ken's mom was sure he had once again neglected to brush.

Tweens can be tough on their teeth. Parents may worry that children in this rough-and-tumble stage will do major damage to their smiles, such as by playing too hard, sneaking forbidden food, or forgoing the toothbrush. At this age, personal hygiene is not a priority, and kids may be so busy with school, sports, and social activities that they don't find time to brush. Children at this age also tend to eat a lot of junk food. Combine the two and you've got a situation ripe for tooth decay. Not surprisingly, many children between the ages of 9 and 12 develop a lot of cavities or begin to have other dental problems.

Milestones

By now your child's teeth have already changed quite a bit, with more baby teeth gone and the permanent incisors in place. You'll probably continue to see some gaps for a while until the rest of the teeth come in. Between ages 9 and 12, your child's primary molars start falling out as the permanent molars begin to emerge. The canines are busy with root formation, and the wisdom teeth are just starting to form.

Caring for Your Child's Teeth

Here are a few tips to help your child get through these years with healthy teeth:

- Encourage your child to keep brushing at least twice a day and flossing daily. At this age, hygiene may not be a priority for most kids, but they do begin to care a lot about how they look. Help your child understand that bad oral hygiene can lead to stains, bad breath, missing teeth, and many other dental problems.
- Set a good example. If you take good care of your teeth, your child will see that good oral hygiene is important to you. Your talks and warnings will be backed up by action and will therefore carry greater weight.
- Have plenty of oral health care supplies on hand. Keep toothbrushes, colored or flavored floss (or easy-to-use plastic flossers), and good-tasting toothpaste in the bathrooms, in the kitchen, and even in the car and your child's backpack for quick use when your preteen is in a hurry.
- Don't buy soda or junk food. Instead, keep lots of fruits and vegetables in the house for snacking.

By what age should my daughter have lost all her baby teeth?

The average age is 11 to 12 years. Between age 9 and 12, she should finally lose her primary upper canine and primary lower second molar. Permanent teeth will generally erupt and push out the baby teeth when their roots are approximately two-thirds formed. If the permanent root development is slow, this delays eruption. Sometimes those baby teeth just won't fall out. By the age of 14 or so, if some baby teeth are still hanging on, it is possible that some of these permanent teeth didn't develop.

If the teen years are approaching, and you're getting worried about teeth that aren't growing, a dental x-ray is the next step. An x-ray can confirm the stage of development of teeth above and below the gum line. If the x-ray shows that some adult teeth are missing, then plan on helping your child keep those baby teeth for as long as possible. Once the rest of the teeth are in, her occlusion (bite) will be stabilized, and you can talk to your child's dentist about options for tooth replacement. Depending on the tooth, you might not have to do anything, and the baby tooth can stay right where it is.

What are twelve-year molars?

As with anything related to growth and development, "twelve-year" molars might come in at age 9, 10, or even 14. These molars are also known as second molars, or teeth numbers 2, 15, 18, and 31. They come in before the wisdom teeth, which are called third molars and are teeth numbers 1, 16, 17, and 32.

When my dentist took x-rays, she said that my son has some extra teeth. What does this mean?

What Is Ankylosis?

Sometimes particularly stubborn primary teeth will not come out due to a condition called ankylosis. The roots of primary teeth are normally attached to the bone through small ligaments, but in ankylosis, they become fused directly to the bone instead. The cause of this condition is not known; it is most likely to happen with lower primary molars. Children who grind their teeth are more likely to experience ankylosis. Because the baby teeth are practically bonded into the jaw bone, it is difficult or impossible for them to extrude on their own or even for them to be extracted by a dentist or an oral surgeon. The permanent teeth may never erupt or may try a different path of eruption and end up in the wrong place.

Sometimes more isn't better, and there's nothing good about having extra teeth, although it isn't uncommon or a big deal. Extra teeth are called supernumary teeth. The most common supernumary tooth is called a mesiodens, which means "middle tooth" because it grows at the midline of the upper jaw. Mesiodens are often malformed nubs but they can look like ordinary teeth. They may be discovered on a routine x-ray or when the teeth are not erupting normally.

Most extra teeth look like regular teeth, with a small crown and a root of some kind. If they form right-side-up and are fairly well formed, they may erupt like normal teeth. If they are upside down, they definitely will not erupt normally. Mesiodens can be problematic and interfere with the normal eruption of the teeth, leading to crowding or impaction. There can even be more than one extra tooth hiding out.

What is the treatment? Many dentists will wait to see if it interferes with the normal eruption of the permanent incisors. If it's not causing an immediate problem, you can wait a bit longer, as long as his dentist is monitoring the situation. If it erupts on its own, then your child's dentist can just extract it like a normal tooth. If it doesn't, and the x-ray shows the potential for problems, then it needs to be surgically removed. Once the offender is removed, the new teeth should erupt in a fairly normal pattern.

How do I know if my child needs braces?

Every child is different, even those in the same family. The best time for getting braces or other dental appliances depends on the type of problem and how severe it is. So the answer really is "it depends." Sometimes early interventions are appropriate while other times, it is necessary to wait until your child's face and jaw are completely developed. In any case, it is important to talk with both your child's dentist and an orthodontist to design the best orthodontic plan for your individual child. (For more information about orthodontics, see chapter 16.)

My daughter's permanent tooth is loose. Should I panic?

If your child is an athlete or accident prone, it's likely you'll encounter a loose permanent tooth at some point. Many people don't realize, however, that a permanent tooth can become loose for lots of reasons, not just injury. Some periodontal disorders destroy the supportive bone around the tooth, for example, and a traumatic occlusion (or bad bite) can cause one tooth to hit before all the other teeth when biting down.

Most traumatic injuries to teeth are from a blow to the face, or a fall that involves the mouth hitting something. If your child's tooth becomes loose from injury, even if you aren't sure if the tooth is permanent, she needs dental care. In most cases, the best treatment is to splint, which means attaching it to the adjacent teeth with a wire, which is bonded to the teeth with a tooth-colored filling material. If adjacent teeth are not available on both sides of the affected tooth, then some type of removable retainer should be used to stabilize the tooth. Periodontal disease so severe that it affects the stability of the tooth is rare in children, but it can happen. Sometimes it is due to a congenital defect in the gum tissue itself, which requires corrective surgery to resolve the problem. Less rare conditions are caused by simple plaque and tartar buildup on teeth that leads to gum disease and results in loose teeth. Aggressive dental work is sometimes needed to restore gum health and salvage those permanent teeth.

The third potential cause for loose permanent teeth is traumatic occlusion, a bad bite, which can usually be fixed easily by a dentist using a process called selective contouring. This involves essentially buffing parts of the enamel to even out the bite, so that all teeth come together at the same time.

> *A Field Trip to Make You Smile*
>
> Want to learn more about dentistry and dental health or share your newfound toothy enthusiasm with your child? Baltimore, Maryland, is home to the National Museum of Dentistry, part of the Smithsonian Institution. As the nation's official museum of the dental profession, it has on display George Washington's actual teeth, vintage toothpaste commercials, and other interactive exhibits encouraging good oral health habits and celebrating dentistry's past, present, and future. If you can't make it to Baltimore, be on the lookout for their traveling exhibitions, which visit different cities nationwide. For more information or to plan your trip, visit www.dentalmuseum.org.

The Battle against Bad Breath

Preteens are in an awkward stage. As if a full-frontal hormonal attack weren't enough to worry about, bad breath can be one more hurdle to overcome. Also known as halitosis, bad breath is a common problem. If your preteen has halitosis, now is the perfect time to get it under control.

After all, adolescence will be hard enough without having to deal with this social liability.

What causes bad breath?

Many factors contribute to bad breath, also called halitosis. Because bacteria from food particles that remain on or in between the teeth can become rotten and emit a foul smell, poor oral hygiene is the number one cause of bad breath. Regular brushing and flossing can prevent this from happening. Other dental conditions that can contribute to halitosis include gum disease, cavities, dry mouth, and bacteria in the mouth and on the tongue. If bad breath is caused by a dental condition, mouthwash and toothpaste will only mask the odor, not cure it. Bring it up with your child's dentist at the next appointment so that the cause can be treated.

Foods can cause bad breath too. What you eat affects the air you exhale. Certain foods, like the well-known offenders garlic and onions and other strong and spicy tastes, contribute to breath odor. Unfortunately, brushing, flossing, and mouthwash will only mask the smell temporarily, and the odors will continue until the body eliminates the food.

Halitosis can also be a symptom of a medical condition, including stomach infections or infections of the mouth, nose, and throat, such as tonsillitis. Uncontrolled diabetes produces a distinctive smell on the breath. If your child's breath smells acidic, she may have gastroesophageal reflux. Colds can also cause bad breath, especially if accompanied by post-nasal drip. Mouth breathing is common with a cold, drying out the mouth, which can cause the breath to smell. In any case, it is important to rule out any medical or dental problems that may be causing chronic bad breath.

Stinky pits, smelly shoes . . . and now bad breath. Is there anything my son can do?

If you have ruled out dental or medical problems, the following steps can help your child get rid of bad breath for good:

- Brush your teeth and tongue twice a day.
- Floss every day.
- Visit the dentist for regular checkups.
- Eat a healthy and nutritious diet.
- Don't use tobacco products.

Children who wear braces should take extra care in practicing good oral hygiene, because food particles can easily become trapped in the braces.

Plaque might also be to blame for strong-smelling breath. If your child has an extensive buildup of plaque, your child's dentist may recommend using a special antimicrobial mouth rinse to eliminate it. It is essential for preteens to learn the benefits of good oral hygiene, which is key to preventing and eliminating bad breath, along with many other dental problems.

If you're convinced your child's dental hygiene is exemplary, and you can't identify any other reasons for persistent bad breath, a quick trip to your health care provider may be helpful.

Does mouthwash help with bad breath?

Many safe, alcohol-free mouthwashes are available for daily use as part of a good oral hygiene program. Some mouthwashes simply disguise the bad breath smell temporarily. An antibacterial mouthwash may help destroy the bacteria in the mouth that cause the breath to smell bad. If your child has halitosis and at-home methods are not working, ask your child's dentist to recommend an appropriate mouthwash.

Children in this age group still need plenty of support, education, and even some old-fashioned nagging, but they are old enough to start accepting responsibility for their choices and for how those choices affect not only their dental health but their overall health as well.

CHAPTER 10

Teenagers and Young Adults (Ages 13+)

"Don't forget to brush your teeth and put in your retainer, Kaylyn," Anna yelled up the stairs toward her daughter's bedroom door. She sighed. Anna wasn't convinced that Kaylyn brushed her teeth more than once a day, and sometimes she wasn't even sure about that. She suspected her daughter's flossing was haphazard as well. Anna had weathered the early years—battling braces and the occasional tooth crisis—and she hoped there wasn't much else she needed to worry about where her daughter's mouth was concerned.

Many parents are surprised at the number of oral health issues that can arise for their teen children. Even with seeing the dentist every six months and maintaining good oral health habits, teens can encounter new problems, especially with puberty affecting the gums and teeth in multiple ways. A teenager's medications, habits, and overall health can play key roles in short-term and long-term oral health.

Milestones

All (or nearly all) of your teen's permanent teeth should be in now. Since the twelve-year molars come in sometime between 10 and 16 years of age, many teens don't realize they need to reach pretty far back to brush those molars. The four third molars, also known as wisdom teeth, are probably still developing under your teen's gums. These teeth usually break through the gum tissue after the age of 17. Some may only partially erupt, and others may stay completely buried under the tissue. Once these molars come in, the set of thirty-two permanent teeth will be complete, although the muscles of the face and mouth are still growing. The bones of your teen's face and jaws, however, are reaching adult strength and dimensions.

At the Dentist

Your 17-year-old son may cringe in horror at having to sit in a pediatric dentist's waiting room decorated with Thomas the Train or filled with hordes of whining toddlers. Where should teenagers go for dental care? Depending on the practice, pediatric dentists can see adolescents until their 18th or 19th birthdays. Although you can transfer your teen's dental care to an adult dentist before this point, pediatric dentists receive special training to meet the unique needs of teens. After all, adolescents experience significant growth in their faces and jaws, the last of their permanent teeth are coming in, and the teeth that have just come through the gums are especially vulnerable to decay. If your teen can stand the cheesy decor, an experienced pediatric dentist is an ideal oral health care provider.

Parents need to continue to provide teens with twice-a-year checkups, complete with x-rays and cleanings, as well as restorative work as needed. Sealants may be applied to any newly emerged teeth, and dentists will usually provide patient education regarding lifestyle habits and oral hygiene. Your teen's pediatric dentist may make a referral to an oral surgeon if wisdom teeth are a concern, or to an orthodontist if your child has problems related to poor bite or to tooth crowding or spacing.

Caring for Your Teen's Teeth

Although your teen is now responsible for his own oral hygiene, you can still take steps to help him improve it.

- Don't hover. Constantly monitoring may backfire and cause your teen to become less interested in what you want him to do.
- Leave some dental pamphlets on a table where your teen can find them and read them privately.
- Never use a visit to the dentist as punishment, which can create a hard-to-shake aversion to the dentist.
- If poor oral hygiene affects the way your teen looks and smells, let him know. "When you don't brush, the plaque on your teeth looks totally gross and makes your breath smell very bad."
- Parents must practice what they preach, brushing at least twice a day and flossing at least once.

Acne Treatment and Discolored Gums

Talk to your teen's health care provider and dentist if your child is prescribed minocycline (Minocin), a commonly prescribed antibiotic for treating acne. It can cause the gums, teeth, and bone to discolor. Tooth discoloration from minocycline does not always resolve after the medicine is stopped. About 5 percent of long-term users have permanently discolored gums.

How does puberty affect my daughter's teeth?

Puberty usually begins for girls around ages 11 to 13 and boys between 12 and 14, and it is not just about acne and growth spurts. The perils of puberty are particularly hard for girls. Raging hormones can cause swollen gums, especially during their periods, when estrogen increases blood circulation to the gums. Herpes-type lesions and ulcers can also occur, and girls may experience gum sensitivity more often. Menstruation gingivitis typically occurs right before a period and clears up once the period has started.

When Average Isn't Good Enough

Oral hygiene is one area where you want your teenager to do better than average. The average teen brushes her teeth once a day, with girls being more likely than boys to brush more than once daily. Teens are even worse with flossing. Even though flossing helps maintain healthy teeth and gums, only 13 percent of teenagers floss their teeth daily, and half of teens report never flossing.

I don't know exactly what my son eats in a given day, but he's like a bottomless pit. How do I know if what he's eating is hurting his teeth?

You are smart to be concerned about your teen's diet. Teenagers eat, on average, nine or ten times

---

Limit the Damage Done by Sugary Drinks

Share these habits with your teen to help prevent (or at least minimize) the damage to teeth and gums caused by sugary drinks.

- Significantly limit carbonated soft drinks and sweetened liquids (like fruit juice).
- Drink fluoridated water and use toothpaste with fluoride.
- Swish out your mouth with water after drinking something sweet to dilute the sugar and acid.
- Use a straw to keep sugars and acids away from your teeth.

- Throw the cap away so you'll be more likely to finish it up and not continuously sip.
- Never consume soft drinks or juice at bedtime. (The liquid pools in your mouth and coats your tongue and teeth.)
- Read the labels—sweetened drinks usually have sugar (or high-fructose corn syrup) as the first ingredient.

---

a day, which might not be a problem if they are eating carrots and celery sticks. Adolescence is the time of peak bone growth, a time when more nutrient-packed calories are essential to fuel growing bodies and strengthen teeth and bones; however, adolescents tend to load up on soda and sugary, high-carbohydrate foods instead of healthy foods, such as milk, fruits, and vegetables. The worse they eat, the more likely they are to have weaker bone structures, which can be devastating later on.

Acid is another problem for teen teeth. Cheerleaders, for example, often suck on lemons to clear their throats during athletic events. That acid damages the enamel of the teeth and can lead to cavities. Soda is even worse for teeth. People who drink three or more sugary sodas daily have 62 percent more dental decay, fillings, and tooth loss. The phosphoric, citric, tartaric, and carbonic acids in soda break down the tooth enamel around dental sealants and restorations, which compromises your teen's teeth and leads to more extensive dental treatment to prevent total tooth loss. The best way to convince teenagers not to drink colas? Show them photographs of the brownish or yellowish teeth of long-term soda or coffee drinkers. Sports drinks are not an improvement over sodas. They often have as much sugar and acid as soft drinks and are more corrosive to both the enamel and the roots of teeth than either soda or juice.

Why is my daughter suddenly getting canker sores?

Canker sores are no fun. These open, shallow sores in the mouth happen to one in five people, and they usually make their first appearance in adolescence. Canker sores, also known as aphthous ulcers, can occur on the under surface of the tongue and on the inside of the cheeks or lips—the parts of the mouth that can move. Usually the sores appear solo, but sometimes they show up in small clusters. The cause is unknown, although they may be related to stress, food allergies, heredity, even hormones—since women are twice as likely as men to develop them.

Your child's mouth might tingle or burn before the actual sore appears. Soon, a small red bump rises. Then after a day or so, it bursts, leaving an open, shallow white or yellowish wound with a red border. The sores are often painful and can be up to an inch across, although they are usually much smaller. They are not contagious like some other mouth sores, such as cold sores, and can't be spread by sharing food or kissing someone.

Your teen can try these tips to tame canker sore pain:

• Place a wet black tea bag against the sore several times a day. The tannin in the tea may help relieve pain.

• Try over-the-counter medications that contain carbamide peroxide (a combination of peroxide and glycerin), benzocaine, menthol, or eucalyptol to help soothe and numb the area, although they may sting at first.

• Rinse your mouth four times a day with a homemade mixture of 2 ounces of hydrogen peroxide and 2 ounces of water or 4 ounces of water mixed with 1 teaspoon (5 milliliters) of salt and 1 teaspoon of baking soda. Swish and spit, but do not swallow.

• Avoid spicy, acidic, and citrus foods, which may irritate the area—citrus and tomatoes can be particularly bad.

(For more information about conditions of the mouth, tongue, and jaw, refer to chapter 15.)

What are the risks of tongue piercing?

Tongue or lip piercing can create some serious problems. The risks of oral piercings include chipped or cracked teeth, blood clots, and blood poisoning. After all, the mouth contains millions of bacteria, and infection is a common complication of oral piercing. The ultimate danger? Although unlikely, an infection in your child's tongue could cause it to swell large enough to close off her airway. Common symptoms after piercing include pain, swelling, infection, increased flow of saliva, and injuries to gum tissue. Difficult-to-control bleeding or nerve damage can result if a blood vessel or nerve is located in the needle's path. About 20 percent of teens with mouth piercings develop tooth fractures on their front teeth. Often small at first, these fractures go unnoticed until the crack enlarges, which can lead to tooth loss, an expensive and embarrassing problem.

No piercings in the mouth area are completely safe. However, you can set some ground rules for a safer experience. Insist that all piercing tools be disposable, that all other equipment be cleaned in an on-site autoclave to help reduce infection, and that the facility be clean and well maintained. Unclean piercing equipment can cause infections like blood-borne hepatitis. Afterward, the pierced area should be rinsed with a chlorhexidine-based mouthwash several times a day for two weeks. As long as the piercing is in place, teach your teen to avoid playing with the piercing and to clean it regularly. Plaque deposits may form over time on the piercing and should be removed by a dentist.

Your child will probably be asked to remove any oral piercings during dental care visits, because jewelry can blur x-ray images and interfere with dental tools, and numbness following an anesthetic can increase the possibility of chipping teeth with

---

Vampire Veneers?

If your teens are jonesing for the latest in toothy trends, they might beg for vampire veneers to give their canines the distinctive pointy shape of pop culture's devilish grin. The veneers are made from material similar to what's used to bond braces on teeth, so it can be put on and taken off easily without damaging the teeth. At $200 or more, veneers are pricey, but they are safer than tooth jewelry or grills that can wreak havoc on other teeth.

the jewelry. The best bet? Insist that your child keep the jewelry away from her mouth, at least until she's footing her own dental care bill.

Does this jewelry match my teeth?

Although it may be fading in popularity, oral jewelry is still making the rounds in some areas. A dental grill, for example, is oral jewelry that is custom fabricated to fit over the top of the upper or lower front teeth. Grills can be removable or permanently glued onto the teeth. To have the jewelry fit in the mouth, healthy tooth structure may be shaved away.

This removal of healthy tooth structure just for wearing decorative mouth jewelry isn't something you want for your child's teeth.

My daughter's dentist suspects that she has bulimia. How would he know?

A dentist can observe damaging effects on the inside surface of the upper front teeth of patients with eating disorders, especially bulimia, a disease that is prevalent among many adolescents, male and female. A telltale sign is eroded enamel caused by repeated regurgitation of acidic stomach contents. After continuous binging and purging, many of these signs can start to appear in the mouth:

- Smooth and worn backs of upper front teeth from erosion
- Thin and translucent teeth
- Eventual tooth loss
- Upper tooth decay that changes the bite as lower teeth move up into the decaying area
- Tooth sensitivity to cold or heat because a tooth nerve is exposed
- Increased risk of periodontal disease
- Dry mouth
- Swollen salivary glands
- Red and sore tongue

- Minor bruises on the roof of the mouth
- Yellowed backs of teeth

Tooth brushing immediately after vomiting may accelerate tooth enamel erosion. Your child's dentist may recommend counseling and prescribe topical fluoride to prevent further erosion. If left untreated, bulimia can have serious medical effects, such as infertility, kidney infections, urinary tract infections, heart irregularities, and even death. In terms of dental care, eating disorders can lead to complete destruction of all teeth and ultimately the need for dentures.

If you know that your child has an eating disorder, it is important to share that information with her dentist. It may be embarrassing for your child, but the dentist should be able to address it in a compassionate, nonthreatening way. You may wish to call the dentist's office before the appointment and ask to have the information written on your child's chart so that you don't have to talk about it in front of her.

> ### Birth Control Pills and Oral Health
>
> Because oral contraceptives mimic pregnancy, women who take birth control pills often experience the same gum changes as pregnant women do. Additionally, women on birth control pills may be more prone to healing problems after dental procedures and surgeries, including dry socket, a painful condition that can lead to infection. Any antibiotics that your child's dentist may prescribe can also interfere with birth control pills, increasing the chance for unintended pregnancy. If your daughter is taking birth control pills, make sure you let her dentist know.

TABLE 10.1. Mouth Problems Associated with Sexually Transmitted Infections

STI	Type of problem	Location
HIV/AIDS	Candida infection, lesions	Gums, palate, tongue
Venereal warts	Pink lesion	Lips, palate, gums, tongue
Gonorrhea	Tonsillitis, inflammation, ulcers	Mucus membranes
Herpes simplex 1	Blisterlike sores	Lips, gums, palate, tongue
Syphilis	Red and ulcerated areas	Gums

What do sexually transmitted infections have to do with my child's teeth?

Teens are becoming sexually active at younger ages and with more partners than in generations before. As a result, they are more vulnerable to sexually transmitted infections, which can lead to various oral health problems. If your child has been diagnosed with such an infection, let your child's dentist know.

How does smoking affect oral health?

Warnings about the health risks of cigarettes probably won't do much to deter teens from smoking. However, some of the potential side effects might be effective in helping an image-conscious teenager reconsider. After all, cigarettes cause bad breath, stained teeth, tooth loss, shrinking gums, mouth sores, decreased senses of taste and smell, poor healing of mouth sores, and hairy tongue leukoplakia, which is as ugly as it sounds. (It is a threadlike irritation on the tongue or cheek that can eventually lead to cancer.) Smokers are also three times more likely than nonsmokers to lose all their teeth.

Even secondhand smoke may cause increased gum disease. Overall, tobacco and healthy teeth just don't mix.

Is chewing tobacco better for teeth than smoking?

Many teens think that smokeless (or chewing) tobacco is somehow safer than cigarette smoking. But that is not true: smokeless tobacco is just as dangerous. It has a higher nicotine concentration than cigarettes and can lead to oral cancer, such as of the gums and lower lips, kidney disease, and strokes.

Chewing tobacco is also cured in sugar, so people who frequently chew tobacco generally have severe tooth decay. This form of tobacco is acidic and tends to erode the surface of the teeth. The erosion process creates a microscopically rough surface on the enamel, allowing stains to

---

Serious Risks Associated with Tobacco Use

- Mouth, tongue, and throat cancer
- Cancer in the esophagus
- Stomach cancer
- Pancreatic cancer
- Increased risk of heart disease, heart attacks, and stroke
- Addiction to nicotine
- Leukoplakia (white sores in the mouth that can become cancer)

- Receding gums (gums slowly shrink from around the teeth)
- Bone loss around the roots of the teeth
- Abrasion (scratching and wearing down) of teeth
- Tooth loss
- Stained teeth (sometimes permanently)
- Bad breath

---

appear and making it difficult to brush away food. Dark brown tobacco juice not only stains the surface of the enamel but also penetrates into the nooks and crannies etched into the surface by the acid. This means that the staining becomes permanent. Smokeless tobacco can also irritate the gums. Once the gums become irritated, they begin to whiten and recede. As the gums recede, the roots of the teeth are exposed, putting the teeth in danger of falling out.

How can I encourage good oral health habits while my son is off at college?

It may sound silly, but use those care packages to send along extra oral health care products. Extra packs of flossers, new toothbrushes, and sugarless gum can be just what a busy college student needs. You could also gently remind your son that red wine can turn teeth yellow and that beer, with its acidic properties, can damage his smile. The other problem with beer is that it contains dehydrating alcohol, causing beer drinkers to produce less saliva. Saliva helps protect teeth from decay (the key word here being "helps"). So after a night on the town, brushing his teeth is still a good idea. Ask your dentist to recommend a dentist in the area,

> **Protect That Smile in the Car**
>
> Sometimes teens and young adults need gentle reminders about safe driving. Let your teen know that another good reason to buckle up in the car is that a seatbelt and shoulder harness can keep his face (and teeth) from striking the steering wheel, the dashboard, or the windshield during minor accidents.

so that your student will be prepared if any dental problems arise.

Our daughter just aged out of our dental insurance. What should she do for her oral health care now?

This is one case where money spent on prevention is money well spent. If you have time to plan before her policy expires, make sure to get in a thorough cleaning and exam with her dentist and take care of potential problems like cavities or gingivitis. Left untreated, small problems can turn expensive quickly.

Preventive measures, like dental sealants, may be a worthwhile investment, even if they aren't covered by insurance, because dental sealants cost about $35 to $60 per tooth, and fillings can cost $150 to $200 each. Of course, practicing excellent oral hygiene, avoiding sweet and sticky foods, and eliminating sodas from her diet will also help keep her teeth healthy and strong.

A Career to Consider?

If your teenager is interested in medicine, she might want to consider dentistry. The median annual wage of a salaried general dentist is about $152,000. Currently, about six hundred to eight hundred more dentists enter the profession than retire from it each year, but starting around 2014, as the baby boomer dentists, who graduated in larger classes, start to retire, the number of practicing dentists will decline while the U.S. population continues to grow. More dental hygienists and dental assistants are also needed. For further information about dentistry as a career, visit the American Dental Education Association Web site at www.adea.org.

CHAPTER 11

Children with Special Health Needs

"I know I should take John to the dentist," Tim told his dad. "But frankly, with his autism, just going to the grocery store can be exhausting. We have been putting off the dentist because he gets overwhelmed so easily, and I can just imagine how he will react. I don't think it's a problem as long as he doesn't complain about his teeth hurting, and we brush and floss his teeth well at home. Maybe in a few years he'll be better able to handle it. Or maybe we both will."

"I don't know," said Tim's dad. "It seems like the longer you don't go, the more likely you'll have problems. But I understand. He doesn't handle new situations well."

Taking care of the oral health of children with special needs can be challenging for everyone—dentists, caregivers, and children. Whether your child has emotional, cognitive, or physical disability or a serious medical condition, he still needs appropriate dental care. The American Academy of Pediatric Dentistry recommends that all children, including those with special health care needs, see a dentist six months after the first tooth comes in, and no later than twelve months after. The AAPD also recommends that children see a dentist for ongoing care at least every six months, depending on the needs of the child.

Caring for Your Child's Specific Needs

Many physical and cognitive disorders are associated with specific dental problems. For example, children with physical disabilities such as cerebral palsy, spina bifida, or muscular dystrophy may have related mouth or dental problems, or they may simply need assistance getting in and out of the dental chair. Other children require adaptive equipment, and some need education in adapting oral health care to their physical abilities to help them better care for their own teeth.

Cognitive or mental health disorders, such as ADHD or autism spectrum disorders (including Asperger syndrome) may heighten a child's anxiety at the thought of going to the dentist or make it difficult to cope with or understand the dental office environment. Complex medical

---

Common Dental Problems in Children with Disabilities

- *Delayed, accelerated, or inconsistent tooth eruption* can occur in children with growth disturbances. Eruption depends on genetics, growth of the jaw, muscular action, and other factors. Children with Down syndrome may show delays of up to two years.
- *Malocclusion* (a poor fit between the upper and lower teeth) and crowding of teeth occur frequently in children with developmental disorders, craniofacial abnormalities, and cognitive disabilities. It is often caused by muscle dysfunction, particularly in people with cerebral palsy. Malocclusion is especially important to understand because teeth that are crowded or out of alignment are more difficult to keep clean, contributing to periodontal disease and tooth decay.
- *Tooth anomalies* are variations in the number, size, and shape of teeth. Children with Down syndrome, oral clefts, ectodermal dysplasia, or other conditions may experience congenitally missing, extra, or malformed teeth.
- *Bruxism,* the habitual grinding of teeth, is common in children with cerebral palsy or severe intellectual disability. In extreme cases, bruxism leads to tooth abrasion and flat biting surfaces.
- *Trauma to the face and mouth* as well as oral infections occur more frequently in people who have cognitive disability, seizures, abnormal protective reflexes, or muscle incoordination.
- *Early, severe periodontal (gum) disease* can occur in children with impaired immune systems or connective tissue disorders and inadequate oral hygiene. Additionally, some medications contribute to gingival overgrowth.

problems in children, such as cardiac defects, HIV/AIDS, or cancer, may mean taking extra precautions before or during dental procedures.

Daily oral health care for all children is as important as their overall health care. Taking into account children's particular needs is essential to ensuring that their dental needs are successfully met, helping them avoid pain, tooth loss, and low self-esteem. Providing this care sometimes takes planning, time, and the willingness and ability to adapt oral health care to a child's physical, mental, and behavioral needs and abilities.

Caring for Your Child's Teeth at Home

One of the best ways to prepare for a successful dental visit is to maintain a regular pattern of frequent oral health care at home. Children need a daily routine of care for their teeth and gums to stay healthy. Many children can be taught how to brush, rinse, and floss independently. Some children will need continued supervision through adulthood, and others need to have dental hygiene performed for them. Every child, regardless of ability, will benefit from this routine activity becoming a standard part of everyday life.

You will face many of the same challenges the dentist does when teaching and providing your child's oral care. The following tips can help you maintain a lifetime of good oral care that works well for you and your child.

- Choose a comfortable location to take care of your child's teeth—somewhere that works for both of you.
- Maintain a consistent and predictable routine for taking care of teeth—same place, same time, same steps—so that your child knows what to expect and gets used to caring for her teeth.
- Get everything ready in advance, including towels, mirror, cup, toothbrush, floss or flosser, toothpaste, and any rinses and cotton swabs you will need.
- Build trust, take it slow, and give lots of positive feedback to reinforce good behavior.
- Make the experience fun for your child by using music, books, toys, puppets, or stuffed animals.

- Keep track of what works, what doesn't, and what questions to ask your child's dentist. Also, note any specific fears or anxieties that don't seem to go away so you can work with your child's dentist on a solution.

  - Don't give up! Remember good oral care is critical for all children and should never be neglected.

> **Pick Your Battles**
>
> Ideally, you would brush your child's teeth at least twice a day. However, if you can only brush your child's teeth once a day, brush before bedtime so that teeth-destroying plaque doesn't sit overnight.

Are there specialized oral care products for children with special needs?

You may need to adapt oral care products to make them work best for your child. For example, if she uses a strap to hold other utensils, she may find it helpful to use the same strap to hold the toothbrush. Some people use a rubber band to hold the brush in place by looping the band over the toothbrush and sliding the hand between the band and the brush. Cutting a slit in a tennis ball and sliding it onto the toothbrush handle can make the brush easier to grasp. Attaching a bicycle grip, pencil grip, or foam tubing to the handle provides a better grip. Other toothbrush options, such as an electric toothbrush, may or may not work for your child. Like most young children, kids with special needs often need a parent's help to floss their teeth, but child-friendly plastic flossers may help them floss on their own.

Taking Your Child to the Dentist

Are pediatric dentists prepared to care for children who have special needs?

Providing oral health care for children with disabilities requires specialized knowledge, increased awareness and attention, and adaptive and accommodative measures beyond what are considered routine. Pediatric dentists often receive training in providing this kind of care, but not every pediatric dentist is comfortable working with children who have special health care needs. Some family practice dentists are experienced and comfortable working with children who face a range of challenges.

Ask for referrals from your child's physician, your family's dentist, or from another parent of a child with a similar diagnosis. Although rare, dentists with mobile dental units in some large urban areas provide dental care in schools, therapeutic settings, and even homes.

For more information about dentistry options for your child, visit the Special Care Dentistry Association at www.scdaonline.org.

Will my child's treatment be different from what other children receive?

Providing oral care for children with special health care needs should generally follow the same standards of practice used with all children. Much of what happens in an ordinary dental visit will still occur. However, depending on your child's specific needs, visits may be more frequent or may require some extra personal attention, accommodations, or modifications. Most important, your child's dentist needs to know about all physical and medical conditions, medications, allergies, emotional issues, and behaviors that will require special attention. If your child sees several specialists, provide the dentist with a list of all other doctors and therapists, along with their contact information and the reason your child is seeing them, when you fill out the initial paperwork.

Talk with your child's primary health care provider before you plan your dental visit. The dentist may need to consult with your child's primary care provider before starting any dental care, especially when a child is taking medications, has a history of allergies, or has conditions related to the heart, lungs, immune system, or diabetes. Children with medically complex care may need their dental work performed in a local hospital. Some children will need to take a course of antibiotics before dental visits.

I'm not sure how my child will react when she gets to the dentist. How do I prepare her?

A "get acquainted" visit with no treatment provided might help. Your daughter can meet the dental team, sit in the dental chair if she wishes, check out the dental instruments, and receive instructions on how to brush and floss. Such a visit can go a long way toward making dental appointments easier. You could also play "going to the dentist" with your child and take turns being the patient and the dentist. Talk about what will happen at the visit, remembering the importance of positive language.

The Center for Children with Special Needs offers a colorful story page, "A Visit to the Dentist," that you can print out and use to prepare your child: http://cshcn.org/sites/default/files/webfm/file/AVisittotheDentist.pdf

What can I do to make sure my child's dental visits are less stressful for everyone?

• See if your child can have the first or last appointment of the day or a time when the office is likely to be less busy.

• Ask if the dental office can mail or e-mail paperwork for you to fill out at home before the visit to minimize your waiting time.

• Find out whether your child can be treated in a private or semiprivate room.

• If your child feels uncomfortable around crowds or new places, wait outside or in your car before the appointment. You can ask the staff to call your cell phone when they are ready for your child.

• Bring a comfort item, such as a favorite toy, stuffed animal, or blanket, if you think it will help your child respond better.

• Ask if you can hold your child's hand or at least sit nearby.

• Make appointments short whenever possible, providing only the treatment that your child can tolerate.

Tell, Show, Do

Many children, including children with special needs, understand much more than they can communicate, which is why many dentists and hygienists use the Tell, Show, Do method. First, they tell the child what they about to do with a dental instrument before starting. Then they show on a model or on their hands what the instrument will do. This is especially important for instruments that make vibrations or sounds. Once the child is comfortable with it, the dentist or hygienist gets the child's permission to do, then slowly introduces the instrument into the patient's mouth. When dental care is handled this way, most children will comply and may even have fun with it.

• Praise and reinforce good behavior and try to end each appointment on a good note.

• Call your child's dentist before the appointment if you have questions about behavioral management during treatment or sedation so that you arrive with a plan.

How can I make sure the dentist meets my child's specific needs?

You are the expert on your child's needs. You know his strengths and challenges, and you will need to communicate clearly with the dental office staff about how best to meet those challenges. Open and honest communication is the key to creating a successful long-term relationship and positive experiences for your child.

Following are some ideas for managing common types of impairments—physical and mobility; vision; hearing; and cognitive.

PHYSICAL AND MOBILITY IMPAIRMENTS

Children with physical and mobility impairments need accommodations to make sure their bodies are comfortable while they receive oral care. As a parent, you will want to know about the office's accessibility, including parking and bathrooms. Also, think about how your child will be transferred to and from the dental chair as gently as possible as well as how to help her keep her mouth open. Determine in advance what modifications might help the dental visit go smoothly for your child. These may include pads or pillows, mouth props, or other supportive devices to help position your child appropriately. Never force her limbs, back, jaw, or neck into an unnatural position. Instead, encourage the dental staff to adjust the chair and move the instruments. In some cases, the dentist and hygienist will need to adjust their positioning to provide care.

VISION IMPAIRMENTS

If your child has difficulty seeing, dental staff will need to help him navigate around the office using his other senses. It is often helpful to minimize background noises, such as music or other office noise, so your child can hear everything clearly. Dental staff should also introduce themselves and ask permission before starting any dental treatments. Encourage the staff to address your child by name while facing him as they work and to describe aloud what they are doing. Sometimes children like to feel the tools before they are used in their mouths. It is important for the dental staff to periodically stop and ask your child if he has any questions or concerns.

HEARING IMPAIRMENTS

Children who are deaf or hard of hearing also need special attention at the dentist. A child who uses sign language may need to have her parent in the room to help communicate, although it is important that dental staff always face the child and talk directly to her instead of only "through" the parent or other caregiver. If your child can read lips, encourage the staff to face her when speaking, using a normal cadence and tone, and to be sure to remove their face masks or wear clear face shields. If your child wears hearing aids, she may need to remove them or turn them off. Ask your child's dentist if the treatments will involve any loud noises or vibrations so that you can prepare your child. Also encourage the use of creative communication. For example, the dental staff can tap once before putting something in your child's mouth, tap twice before starting the suction, and so on. They can also use flash cards or pictures to communicate or educate.

COGNITIVE IMPAIRMENTS

Cognitive impairments can occur in children due to a wide range of conditions, including fragile X syndrome, Down syndrome, and fetal alcohol syndrome. Mental capabilities vary in children with developmental disorders and influence how well they can follow directions in the dental office and at home. Talk with your child's health care providers about his ability to communicate and to understand instructions, as well as how his abilities might affect oral health care. Be receptive to their thoughts and ideas on how to make the experience a success.

For more information about specific special needs and oral health care, contact the Oklahoma Association of Community Action Agencies at www.okacaa.org for their free publication *Oral Health Care for Children with Special Health Care Needs*.

My child has autism, and I am afraid he won't be able to tolerate a dental visit. What can I do to make it easier?

A minor difference in your son's routine may make him feel like the world is going to end. Your child may have a debilitating fear of change and new experiences. Going to a new store can be a challenge, not to mention a medical facility. What can you do? If your child has a set of flip cards to help him with his daily schedule, create a special flip card that shows a toothbrush and floss. Teach your child that he will see this card in the morning and at night. When it's time to visit the dentist, introduce a special flip card that shows a dentist (or maybe a picture of the dental office) and place it in his flip schedule at the appropriate time. Children with autism often depend on the consistency of a regular daily structure.

Because the dentist's office is a strange environment with unfamiliar people, patients who have autism are likely to find the entire experience confusing. One of the best approaches for some children is a slow acclimation process, although it's time consuming. Many children, even those without specific diagnoses or challenges, need to have new experiences explained to them first. Preparation can be the key to whether a child accepts new information or a new experience with enthusiasm or fear. For children with autism or sensory disorder, this is even more true. With several acclimation visits before a new patient exam, your child might accomplish much more than he or you ever thought possible.

Find out if you can take a tour or play in the playroom. Ask if your child can simply sit in the exam chair, then pick out a toy favor and go home. Come back a second or third time and work toward completing the full exam.

Unfamiliar or strong smells send my daughter into a tailspin. Are there ways to help the staff prepare for her sensory issues?

Sensory issues can interrupt treatment. Children with Asperger syndrome or autism are among those who may exhibit unusual sensitivity to sensory stimuli, such as sound, bright colors, and touch. Reactions vary: some children may overreact to noise and touch, while exposure to pain and heat may not provoke much response at all. Talk to the dental staff about how to minimize overly strong responses. Schedule each visit at the same appointment time with the same dentist and, if possible, arrange for the same staff members to work with your child. The familiarity can help make dental treatment seem less threatening. Work with the dental office to minimize distractions and reduce unnecessary sights, sounds, odors, or other stimuli that might be disruptive. Request a dental chair that is somewhat secluded instead of one in the middle of a busy office. Ask if staff can lower ambient light and play soft music, or if your child can wear headphones. Some children who are hypersensitive to the sound of dental instruments may find that headphones minimize their distress. Allow time for your child to adjust and become desensitized to the noise of the office.

> ### Be Aware of Aversions
>
> An aversion is a strong dislike of something, such as a strong taste or particular textures. Children can develop oral aversions after experiencing trauma of any kind to their mouths such as cleft lip or palate, use of ventilator or feeding tubes, or oral or facial surgery or trauma. Some children have an aversion to touch and dislike being handled by dental staff. This can make oral care in a regular dental office challenging, or even impossible. It is important to determine the level of any aversions your child has before proceeding with her care. Before any appointment, talk with your child's dentist about how dental staff should approach your child to gain the most cooperation.

Talk to your child's dentist about her level of tolerance. Every child is different. Encourage the staff to record in your child's chart what works for her, so everyone is prepared for next time.

My son has a seizure disorder. What can I do to keep him safe during dental treatments?

Visiting the dentist is very important for children who have seizures. Seizures themselves, as well as the medications taken for them, can put your child at greater risk for chipped or broken teeth, gum disease, and dry mouth. Because seizures can occur spontaneously and can be triggered by stimuli, such as certain sounds or sudden movements, it is critical to work with your child's dentist to ensure a safe and effective visit. First, set up a pre-appointment interview with the dental staff to discuss your child's medical history and seizure triggers (if any) and how to handle a seizure if your child has one during his appointment. Being prepared to manage a seizure is the most important factor in keeping your child safe. Talk to your health care provider about the most appropriate time to take the anti-seizure medication prior to the dental appointment. Ask the dental staff to attach dental floss to instruments before dental treatment begins so that they can be quickly removed if needed. According to the publication *Oral Health Care for Children with Special Health Care Needs*, developed by the Oklahoma Developmental Disabilities Council, if a child has a seizure, dental staff should do the following:

Dental Care for Cleft Lip or Palate

A child with a cleft lip or palate requires the same regular preventive and restorative care as a child without a cleft. Many children with clefts have special problems related to missing, malformed, or malpositioned teeth, and they usually require early evaluation by a dentist who is familiar with the needs of a child with a cleft. Dental treatments may include earlier dental care, orthodontics, or coordinated prosthodontic and dental-surgical care. For more information, visit the Cleft Palate Foundation Web site at www.cleftline.org.

- Remove instruments from the mouth and clear the area around the chair.
- Do not insert any objects between the child's teeth.
- Stay with the child, turning him to one side and monitoring his airway until the seizure passes. A staff person should go get you if you are not present, but not if this means leaving your child alone.

• Once the seizure is over, staff should comfort your child and make sure he understands that he is okay and that the treatment will go on or stop, depending on what you and the dentist decide.

My daughter can't always control the muscles in her mouth and throat. Is there any point in her even going to the dentist?

Yes! The appointment might take longer than usual, but you and the dental staff can do more than you might think to minimize problems and keep your child as comfortable as possible. Neuromuscular disorders, such as muscular dystrophy, affect the nerves that control voluntary muscles. Some people with neuromuscular disorders have persistently rigid or loose masticatory muscles, the muscles used in chewing. Others have drooling, gagging, biting, and swallowing problems that complicate oral care. If your child has a problem with gagging, schedule an early morning appointment, before she eats or drinks anything. Help minimize the gag reflex by placing her chin in a neutral or downward position. If she has swallowing problems, tilt her head slightly to one side and place her body in a more upright position. Dental instruments should be slowly placed in the mouth. Suction can be used as frequently as tolerated.

If your child has uncontrolled body movements, tell the dental staff not to force her limbs into unnatural positions but to allow her to settle comfortably in the chair. It is important for the staff not to attempt to stop movements, although firm, gentle pressure can calm a shaking limb.

Controlling the Gag Reflex

Some children have a sensitive, overactive, or high gag reflex, making it difficult to put anything in their mouths. Something as simple as certain foods or a toothbrush can cause a child to gag, cough uncontrollably, or even vomit. As a result, the child becomes more upset and distressed. The key is to get your child to relax in order to desensitize this reaction. Try to get him to remain calm and to breathe through his nose. While in a low-stress environment, such as at home, get your child to practice controlling his gag reflex while doing ordinary tasks like eating and brushing. Dentists can give medications that further relieve this reflex during dental visits. Most overactive gag reflexes can be overcome with patience and practice, and many children improve at controlling it as they get older. As frustrating as it may be, don't let an overactive gag reflex prevent your child from getting good oral care.

The staff can try to anticipate and work around movements, keeping equipment out of range of your child's limbs. They should also tone down lights and attempt to prevent sudden unexpected sounds.

My daughter is in a wheelchair. Does she need to be moved to the dental chair?

Performing examinations and some preventive care with children in their wheelchairs is sometimes preferable to transferring the child, particularly if the wheelchair can be adjusted. If your child needs to be transferred, ideally the wheelchair should fit parallel to the dental chair. Transfers are more difficult if the area is too crowded to align the chairs. If the dental chair does not have movable armrests, lifting your child into the chair could be a problem, especially if she wears leg or back braces.

When first choosing a dentist for your child, find out if the office, parking lot, and x-ray equipment are accessible to children in wheelchairs. Also ask about the policy on transferring children. If staff members prefer to do the transfer themselves, you will want to make sure they have received appropriate training and have a transfer board if needed.

You can also practice the "knee to knee position" at home. This is a common position for providing dental care for small children or children in wheelchairs. In this position, you and the dentist sit facing each other, with knees touching. You hold your child facing toward you and then lay her back down across your legs with her head cradled in the dentist's lap.

Antibiotic Prophylaxis

Before some dental treatments, people who have certain heart conditions, including congenital heart conditions (present since birth), and people who have artificial joints need to take antibiotics. This is called antibiotic prophylaxis, meaning the antibiotics are meant to prevent infection, not treat one. For more information about the specific recommendations, check with the American Heart Association (www.heart.org) or the American Academy of Orthopedic Surgeons (www.aaos.org) and discuss with your child's dentist how these recommendations might affect your child.

What if my child simply will not allow the dentist to perform a procedure?

First of all, you and the dental team should pay careful attention to preparing your child for the visit, clearly explaining what is happening and being aware of early signs and clues about how your child is responding. When a child is unable or unwilling to cooperate with oral care, and all methods of behavioral management have been tried without success, the next step to consider is some form of physical stabilization. Stabilization methods include sedation, anesthesia, and physical restraints. Each method has advantages and risks and should always be carefully discussed with the dentist to ensure the safety of both your child and the dental staff. Every visit is different, and children change, so the methods may need to be modified each time your child sees the dentist. For instance, after several dental experiences, a child who required sedation may no longer need it.

Many children with special needs do well with sedation dentistry (sometimes called conscious sedation). To ensure good dental health as well as safety, children are given medication to help them relax or even sleep through the treatments. These medications can be given orally, by a shot, or as a gas that is inhaled through a mask. Even though your child becomes very relaxed, his brain is not altered, and he should be able to remember the experience, hopefully as a calm and positive one.

Occasionally, general anesthesia is needed, especially if the dental work is done in a hospital setting or involves surgery. To ensure safety, laws regulate who can administer general anesthesia, including for dental patients. With this form of sedation, your child is asleep and will not be aware of what's happening. Although it eliminates fear and anxiety, there is a risk of reaction to the anesthesia as there is with all medications. It is important to discuss these risks, and any other concerns you might have, with your child's dentist and perhaps his pediatrician too.

Very rarely, physical restraints are recommended, which can be traumatic, increasing stress levels and sometimes risking injury, which can influence how children view the dentist for the rest of their lives. There may be times, however, when restraints are the only option. Always discuss with your child's dentist beforehand, in detail, what type of restraint will be used, how it will be used, duration of use, both risks and benefits of the proposed methods, and whether there are any other options. Dentists should strive to use the least restrictive, yet safest and most effective methods.

Reward Work Well Done

Whenever your child succeeds at something challenging, provide praise and encouragement. This includes a completed dental visit. A hug, special time with Mom or Dad, or a high five can all go a long way toward leaving your child with a memory of a positive dental experience.

PART III

Dental and Oral Health Problems

CHAPTER 12

Tooth Decay

Keeping teeth healthy, white, and shiny is harder than it seems. Whether you're protecting your child's teeth against bumps and falls, keeping track of which teeth come in when, or being a toothbrush warrior while battling an uncooperative 4-year-old, you also need to be prepared for potential problems, starting with the outside of those pearly whites. Did we say pearly whites? Let's be clear: no one outside of Hollywood truly has pearly white teeth. Normal, healthy tooth color ranges from palest yellow to grayish white. And it all boils down to your enamel.

Enamel Basics

Enamel is the hard outer surface layer of teeth that protects against tooth decay. Tooth enamel is in fact the hardest mineral substance in the body, stronger even than bone. Enamel helps protect teeth from all the chewing, biting, crunching, and grinding they do. It also insulates the teeth from potentially painful temperatures and chemicals. Enamel ranges in thickness from about 0.5 to 2.5 millimeters.

Despite its strength, enamel can chip and crack. Everyday acids that develop from certain foods and drinks, particularly those that contain sugar or starch, can put enamel at risk. These acids soften the tooth surface. Plaque bacteria produce acids that can weaken and destroy the enamel, too. Unlike a broken bone that can be repaired by the body, once a tooth chips or breaks, the damage is done forever. Because enamel has no living cells, the body cannot repair it. Once it is gone, it's gone for good. Without the protection of enamel, teeth are vulnerable to a host of new problems.

What causes enamel problems?

When acidic content hits the tooth surface, it erodes the enamel. Erosion can be caused by something as simple as excessive consumption of soft drinks or fruit drinks. Soft drinks have high levels of phosphoric and citric acids, and some acids in fruit drinks are more erosive than battery acid. Erosion can be caused by any of the following:

- Diets high in sugar and starches
- Dry mouth or low salivary flow
- Acid reflux disease (or GERD)
- Gastrointestinal problems
- Medications (such as aspirin, antihistamines, and some vitamins or antibiotics)
- Medical conditions and illnesses, especially involving compromised immune systems or numerous fevers
- Frequent vomiting—in eating disorders, for example
- Any combination of friction, wear and tear, stress, and corrosion

How can I protect the enamel on my son's teeth?

First, your child should use toothpaste that contains fluoride. Numerous scientific studies over the past fifty years have proven the benefit of fluoride in strengthening and protecting tooth enamel against daily acid attacks.

Second, your child should brush and floss regularly. Dentists recommend tooth brushing at least twice a day, along with daily flossing, to help promote oral health.

Third, he should see a dentist every six months for regular checkups and cleaning. Talk to his dentist about daily fluoride treatments for your child if you have a family history of enamel erosion or cavities. In addition, ask your child's dentist if sealants may help prevent enamel erosion and tooth decay in your child's mouth.

You can also try the following:

- Eliminate sodas and juices and other highly acidic foods and drinks from your child's diet. If he does eat or drink an acidic food, have your child rinse his mouth out right away with water.
- Ask your child to use a straw when drinking. The straw pushes the liquid to the back of the mouth, so it comes into contact with fewer teeth.
- Monitor your child's snacks. Snacking throughout the day increases the chance of tooth decay. The more you snack, the longer your mouth is filled with sugar and starches, which feed the cavity-causing bacteria. If your child does snack, have him rinse his mouth and brush his teeth afterward.
- Offer sugar-free gum between meals. Chewing gum boosts saliva production up to ten times the normal flow, which helps strengthen teeth. Select sugar-free gum with xylitol, which has also been shown to benefit teeth.
- Make sure you child drinks plenty of water throughout the day.

Enamel in Clinical Terms

Your child's dentist may refer to the tooth changes that affect enamel using clinical terms like these:

- Attrition. This is natural tooth-to-tooth friction that happens when your child clenches or grinds her teeth (bruxism), which often occurs involuntarily during sleep.
- Abrasion. This is physical wear and tear of the tooth surface, which happens with brushing teeth too hard, improper flossing, biting on hard objects (such as fingernails, bottle caps, or pens), or chewing tobacco.
- Abfraction. This term refers to stress fractures in the tooth, such as cracks from flexing or bending it.

What are the signs of enamel erosion?

The signs of enamel erosion progress through these stages:

1. Discoloration. As the enamel erodes and more dentin is exposed, the teeth become yellow.
2. Sensitivity. Because the enamel protects the teeth, certain foods and temperatures may cause a twinge of pain in the early stage of enamel erosion.

In later stages of enamel erosion, as the dentin becomes even more exposed, teeth will become extremely sensitive and painful.

3. Transparency. The front teeth might begin to look transparent, especially at the edges, and develop a smooth or shiny appearance.

4. Cracking and chipping. The edges of teeth become more rough, irregular, and jagged as enamel erodes, which is especially noticeable as you run your tongue over them. Sometimes the teeth have a rounded look or appear shorter.

How is enamel loss treated?

Treatment of tooth enamel loss depends on what's causing it. Sometimes tooth bonding is used to protect the tooth and improve its appearance. If the enamel loss is significant, your child's dentist may recommend covering the tooth with a crown. The crown may protect the tooth from further decay. A lack of enamel in children should be evaluated by a dentist to identify the cause and to decide what can be done about it. If left unmonitored or untreated, enamel loss can lead to severe tooth sensitivity and cavities.

Tooth Decay

Tooth decay is damage to teeth that is permanent and irreversible in nearly all cases. Tooth decay is similar to tooth erosion. Both processes involve damage to the protective enamel of teeth. Tooth erosion typically occurs when we expose our teeth to a large quantity of acid, mostly through foods or drinks. Erosion causes the enamel to soften and eventually dissolve away, providing a direct path for bacteria to enter the teeth. Once inside this protective barrier, the bacteria continue to release acid, which works to destroy the entire tooth.

What are dental plaque, calculus, and tartar?

Dental plaque is a sticky mass of bacteria and other organic material that accumulates on the tooth's surface. Bacteria produce adhesive chemicals called mucopolysaccharides, which produces a slimy film on the teeth, also called biofilm. Although plaque cannot be rinsed off, it can be removed by brushing and flossing. The longer it remains on teeth, the greater the risks of gum disease. It is also responsible for bad breath. Diets rich in soft, sticky, carbohydrate foods with high sugar content encourage plaque formation.

Plaque forms more easily in certain places, such as

- cracks, pits, or grooves in the back teeth
- between teeth
- around dental fillings or bridgework
- near the gum line

If plaque is not removed, it can harden to form calculus, also called tartar. Basically, tartar is petrified plaque, and it can't be brushed off. It can only be removed by a dentist or dental hygienist. Older children, who have had more time for plaque to build up, are more likely than younger children to have calculus.

What are dental caries?

Dental caries is the medical term for a disease or process that causes tooth decay, such as the process of plaque causing cavities. Some of the bacteria in plaque continue to convert the sugar and carbohydrates (starches) in the foods we eat into acids. These acids dissolve minerals in the surface of the tooth, eroding the enamel or creating pits in it that are too small to see at first. Over time, these pits get larger, creating cavities.

Cavity damage can occur wherever the tooth is exposed to plaque and acid. This includes the hard outer enamel on the tooth crown as well as parts of the root. Once decay penetrates the protective enamel, it can enter

---

Lemons and Ice

Almost everyone has some type of bad habit. A few seemingly innocent habits (often starting in childhood) can wreak havoc on teeth. Sucking on lemons, for example, can erode enamel. Over time, the teeth will become more susceptible to cavities or will develop tiny grooves that lead to chipping or other tooth problems.

Chewing on ice cubes can also be a disaster for your child's teeth. The sudden cold compromises the enamel. In addition, chewing ice can lead to a cracked tooth or make existing fillings expand and contract, rapidly weakening the tooth.

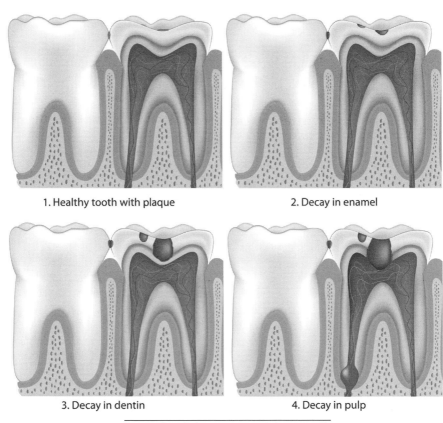

1. Healthy tooth with plaque

2. Decay in enamel

3. Decay in dentin

4. Decay in pulp

Stages of tooth decay. © Can Stock Photo Inc. / alila

the softer, more vulnerable dentin, which is the main body of the tooth. A cavity can even penetrate the soft tooth pulp and the sensitive nerve fibers within it, causing severe pain.

What are the symptoms of tooth decay?

Early tooth decay may not have any symptoms. As the decay eats through the enamel, the tooth becomes sensitive to sweet foods or to hot and cold temperatures. Although no one knows for sure what causes the pain some people get with cavities, theories include:

• Inflammation caused by bacteria

- Exposure of the root surface
- Imbalance of fluid levels in tiny openings inside the dentin

When cavities have been present for a long time but have not been treated, they usually become visible. An ignored cavity will usually look like a dark spot on your child's tooth, although sometimes it's an area lighter than the rest of the tooth, or a hole in the affected tooth. If you notice any of these symptoms in your child's teeth, you should take her to the dentist right away, because an ignored cavity can affect your child's oral and overall health.

How is tooth decay or a cavity diagnosed?

As part of dental exams, whether routine office visits or appointments made because of pain, dentists look for tooth decay. They do this by visually examining the teeth as well as probing them with a tool called an explorer to look for pits and other areas of damage. X-rays might be taken if the dentist suspects hidden cavities.

Does tooth decay always lead to a cavity?

Cavity formation needs two things: dental plaque and dietary sugars. Although these conditions don't always exist, each time they do, some tooth demineralization will occur. Demineralization simply describes the

---

Beware of Baby Kisses!

This may sound hard to believe, but when you give your baby a quick kiss on the lips, nibble on baby toes, or smooch those perfect fingers, those oh-so-sweet touches may be hurting your baby. Tooth decay is actually an infectious disease. The cavity-causing bacteria that are in your mouth transfer easily to your baby's fingers and toes, which often go straight into her mouth. This doesn't mean you can't give kisses, but you might want to avoid kissing those parts that go directly into baby's mouth. But that shouldn't be too difficult. After all, what's more delicious than a perfect baby belly button?

dissolving of mineral content (like calcium compounds) out of the tooth's hard tissues, such as the tooth enamel. A person doesn't develop cavities overnight, because conditions aren't always right for the tooth demineralization process. Over time, however, the cumulative effect of demineralization episodes can result in a cavity forming.

Early tooth decay may be reversed if acid damage is stopped and the tooth is given a chance to repair the damage naturally. Tooth decay that has destroyed enamel cannot be reversed. If left untreated, most cavities will continue to get worse and deeper. With time, the tooth may decay down to the root. The amount of time this erosion takes will vary from person to person. It can take months or years for a cavity to erode to a noticeably painful level.

> **My Grandma Always Said That Our Family Has Soft Teeth. Was She Right?**
>
> Not really. The reason she had bad teeth, and the reason you have cavities, has absolutely nothing to do with having soft teeth. Both the strongest teeth and the weakest are prone to the exact same problem—tooth decay from bacteria. Because tooth decay is an infectious disease, it is one of the most common chronic conditions among children. But there's good news: it is preventable.

Do certain foods cause cavities?

Many different types of foods besides candy can cause tooth decay in children. Foods high in carbohydrates, such as fruits, juices, sodas, crackers, and potato chips, are common culprits. How often the foods are eaten and how long they remain as particles in the mouth affect whether they will lead to tooth decay. Occasional treats are fine, but candy, snacks, and soda can't be the mainstay of your child's diet if you want him to have a healthy smile for a lifetime.

How can I prevent cavities in my child?

You can prevent cavities by reducing the amount of plaque and bacteria in your child's mouth. The best way to do this is by daily brushing and flossing and getting professional dental cleanings twice a year. You can also reduce the amount of acid in your child's mouth by cutting down on the sugary or starchy foods available to him. Your child's mouth will remain acidic for several hours after eating, so snacking or grazing throughout the day is more likely to lead to tooth decay than not eating in between meals. Chewing gum that contains xylitol may help counteract the effects of plaque after eating.

Teeth can also be strengthened with fluoride. A dentist can evaluate your child's risk of cavities and then suggest appropriate fluoride treatments. Permanent molars can be sealed after they erupt. Dentists can also use sealants on molars that have early signs of tooth decay, as long as the decay has not broken through the enamel.

Treating Cavities in Children

The standard treatment for a cavity is to fill the tooth. At a filling appointment, your child's dentist will usually begin with a quick inspection to confirm that the job has to be done. Then a local anesthetic (pain-blocking injection) is used if necessary. If the filling is superficial, a local anesthetic may not be needed. If the cavity extends beyond the enamel or if the preparation will be uncomfortable, however, a local anesthetic is recommended. A topical anesthetic gel may be used first, to lessen the feeling in the gum before injection. If your child is not cooperative, other sedatives, such as nitrous oxide, may be considered to make the whole experience quicker and more tolerable. The dentist will be experienced in giving the anesthetic in the kindest possible way.

The decay is then removed with a drill or hand instruments. The dental assistant then sucks away the water and debris from the drilling, and the dentist fills the cavity, usually with amalgam or composite. Amalgam is a silver-gray material made from silver mixed with copper or other metals to make it more durable. Amalgams are used primarily in molars and premolars, which are not easily seen. Composites look better because they are tooth-colored, so they are used in the front teeth, although it is possible to use them in all teeth for a better appearance. Gold inlay may be used if greater strength is needed, but this is more expensive and not as common as it used to be.

A metal band is sometimes put around the tooth to act as a mold while the filling is placed. After a quick check of the bite, your child's dentist will file down any extra filling material, and that's it. Your child should feel proud of herself for being so brave and making it through the treatment. Make sure to lavish her with praise for a job well done.

If a cavity is large, the remaining tooth may not be able to support the amount of filling material that would be needed to repair it. In this case, the dentist will remove the decay, fill the cavity, and cover the tooth with an artificial crown. Sometimes the part of the tooth you can see remains relatively intact, but there is damage deep inside. In these cases, your child's dentist might recommend a root canal treatment. (For more information about root canals, see chapter 19.)

> **The First Drill**
>
> John Greenwood invented the dental drill in 1790. It was big and heavy, and the dentist had to turn a handle (like using a hand drill for drilling holes in wood) to drill out all the bad bits in the tooth. It was a slow and painful process, so people only went to the dentist when they couldn't stand the pain of a toothache any longer.

How quickly do I need to get my child's cavity filled?

That's a little like asking how long you can wait to call the exterminator about termites in your house. Cavities don't stop growing. Nobody can tell you when cavities will get critical. Getting cavities filled can be uncomfortable for your child and expensive for you, but if the cavity infects the pulp, your child might need a root canal, which can be far more complicated (and expensive) than a filling.

You usually cannot tell how deep or severe a cavity is until it is x-rayed. A small visible cavity on a tooth can be huge and deep when seen on x-ray. Although there is no set "safe" time frame for waiting to have a cavity filled, once the cavity affects the nerve, you won't need an x-ray to tell you how bad it is. The cavity will become painful for your child, requiring an urgent visit to the dentist. Basically, the sooner a cavity is detected and fixed, the easier and cheaper it will be to fix. Without treatment, the tooth may be destroyed by uncontrolled decay.

Some parents opt not to treat cavities because of the cost or other reasons. Although we do not want to recommend not getting a cavity filled, there is some flexibility with this; for example, you don't necessarily need to get every cavity filled immediately every time the dentist finds one. Talk to your child's dentist about how your child's specific risks affect the time frame for treating cavities.

Keep in mind that having cavities increases your child's risk of *more* cavities, for a few reasons:

- The same oral care and dietary habits that led to the erosion of teeth by plaque and acids may continue to cause more decay in other teeth.
- Bacteria tend to stick to fillings more than to smooth unfilled teeth, so areas adjacent to fillings are more likely to be at risk for cavities.
- Cracks or gaps in the fillings may allow bacteria and food to enter the tooth, leading to decay from beneath the filling.

What happens after a filling?

Your child's lip, tongue, and cheek will usually be numb for about 1 to 2 hours. Be watchful so that your child does not accidentally bite her numb cheek, tongue, or lip, or scratch around his nose. Accidental biting can cause the lip, cheek, tongue, or face to swell. If your child feels any discomfort after the numbness wears off, give her the appropriate dosage of acetaminophen (Tylenol) or ibuprofen (Motrin).

After dental treatment, some mild swelling of the lip or cheek and some bruising at the injection site is normal. Swelling can happen quickly, though, so watch your child carefully for the first 1 to 2 hours after the appointment. Time is the best healer of mild swelling. Major swelling could indicate an allergy (although rare) or another reason for concern, so contact your child's health care provider if this occurs. Call 911 or take your child to the emergency room if you believe she is having a medical emergency.

Keep your child on a liquid diet for the first 4 hours and then on a soft diet for the remainder of the day. Soft foods include Jell-O, soups, pasta, eggs, yogurt, pudding, applesauce, soft cheeses, and mashed potatoes. Do not give your child hot foods or foods that have to be chewed. Hard foods

Laser Use in Dentistry

Lasers have been used by dentists since 1994, and many are approved by the Food and Drug Administration for use in dentistry. Although the American Dental Association has yet to give dental lasers the official ADA Seal of Acceptance for meeting its safety and efficacy standards, the ADA is cautiously optimistic about the role of laser technology in the future of dentistry, including with children. Lasers can be used to treat tooth decay or gum disease, to do biopsies or remove lesions, and for endodontics and whitening teeth. Overall, lasers may cause less pain, reduce anxiety about dental treatments, minimize bleeding and swelling, and preserve more healthy tooth during cavity removal. However, dental lasers cannot be used for all dental problems and can be expensive, so they will probably not completely replace traditional dentistry.

and heavy chewing may cause the filling to fracture if your child eats them too soon after the filling is placed.

Can my daughter have drill-less dentistry done instead?

Some dentists offer drill-less dentistry, also called air abrasion and microabrasion, to simply and quickly remove minor tooth decay, superficial stains, and discolorations as well as to prepare a tooth surface for bonding or sealants. The air abrasion instrument works like a mini-sandblaster, using compressed air to spray a fine stream of particles at the tooth surface. As the stream of particles strikes, small bits of decay on the surface of the tooth are removed and suctioned away. Although drill-less dentistry lessens the pain usually experienced with dental procedures, some patients do feel tooth sensitivity. Not all dental offices offer drill-less dentistry, but it is likely to become more widely used, since it is better for treating less serious cases of tooth decay. Drill-less dentistry usually works well for children who have dental fears and only minimal decay.

CHAPTER 13

Gum Disease

Chances are you haven't given much thought to your child's gums, but there's good reason to start, because healthy gums hold and protect your child's precious pearly whites. These pink and spongy structures are an integral part of a healthy mouth. The job description for the gums is simple: adhere to the teeth closely to prevent infection from entering the teeth, or from spreading if it does. Infection that gets past the gum line defense can get to the roots of the teeth or jaw bone and cause serious damage. Gum disease, not old age, is the leading cause of tooth loss.

Develop the habit of regularly checking your child's gums for redness, swelling, or anything else that looks unusual for your child.

Periodontal Disease

Periodontal disease is a chronic bacterial infection that affects the gums and bone supporting the teeth. The word *periodontal* literally means "around the tooth." The disease can affect one tooth or many teeth. It begins when the bacteria in plaque (the sticky, colorless film that constantly forms on teeth) cause the gums to become inflamed. That irritated gum tissue pulls away from the teeth, which allows bacteria to destroy the underlying bone supporting the teeth. Gum disease can occur in your child's baby teeth or permanent teeth.

Gums that have become weakened or recessed provide a pathway for tooth loss. Gum disease can affect anyone, of any age. The types of gum disease most common in children are gingivitis (which causes gums to become red, swollen, and tender and to bleed easily), mild periodontitis (which causes bad breath, pockets between the teeth and gums, loose teeth, and tooth loss), and moderate to advanced periodontitis (which can lead to tooth decay). Periodontal disease actually affects any one or more of the periodontal tissues:

- Gums (also called gingiva), the soft, pink tissue that covers the alveolar bone
- Cementum, a bony layer that covers the lower parts (roots) of the teeth
- Alveolar bone, the bone where the roots of the teeth are embedded
- Periodontal membranes or ligaments, membranes composed of fibers that connect and attach the root of the tooth to the bone

> *The Link between Gum Disease and Other Diseases*
>
> Researchers continue to find associations between periodontal disease and several other serious health problems. So far, studies have linked gum disease in adults to an increase in
>
> - heart disease
> - diabetes
> - dementia
> - rheumatoid arthritis
> - premature birth
>
> Eradicating gum disease early can clearly help prevent long-term health problems.

All periodontal diseases, including gingivitis and periodontitis, are serious and, if untreated, can lead to tooth loss—even in children. Anyone can experience gum disease, but risk factors include genetics, stress, medications, tobacco use, diabetes, poor nutrition, and hormonal changes, often seen in puberty.

What is gingivitis?

Gingivitis is the mildest form of periodontal disease and the most common form in children. In fact, up to 35 percent of children between the ages of 3 and 5 have at least some signs of gingivitis. By the teenage years, the incidence increases to 90 percent. In gingivitis, the gums become red and swollen, and they bleed easily, although there is usually little or no discomfort. Gingivitis is often caused by inadequate oral hygiene. Fortunately, this form of gum disease is both preventable and treatable with good oral care at home and professional dental treatments. Typically, more boys than girls have gingivitis, probably because girls tend to have better oral hygiene habits than boys do, rather than because of any physiological differences. If it is not treated, chronic gingivitis can advance to more serious forms of periodontal disease.

Common symptoms of gingivitis include:

- A change in the color of gums from pink to red or bluish red
- Swelling of the gum margins closest to the teeth
- Blood on the toothbrush during brushing
- Gums that have receded from the base of the teeth
- Chronic bad breath
- Loose permanent teeth
- Open sores on the gums

> **What Color Is Normal for Gums?**
>
> In Caucasian and Hispanic people, gums are typically pink. African Americans have dark pink or reddish gums. There is a wide variation of normal for gum color. What's important is to be aware of color changes. It isn't normal for your child's gum color to change. Red gums may indicate gum infection, and white gums may indicate infection elsewhere in your child's body. (The activity of white cells causes the color change.)

What is gingival hyperplasia?

Often called gingival overgrowth, gingival hyperplasia is a condition where the soft tissues of the gums grow out of control. The most common cause of this overgrowth is a side effect of some medications. Through good oral hygiene, gingival hyperplasia can be controlled but not always prevented. Treatment includes regular dental visits, cleanings, and in some cases surgical repair.

Do bleeding gums always mean gum disease?

Although gum bleeding is a common symptom of gingivitis, it is not necessarily due to gum disease. Mouth injury or trauma, such as a blow to the mouth, insertion of foreign substances, tooth picking, improper brushing, or flossing can cause the gums to bleed. Gums may also be irritated by chemicals and acids in foods, drinks, mouth fresheners, tooth whiteners, or medicines. In rare cases, gum bleeding can be an early sign of leukemia. Any bleeding from the gums warrants a call to the dentist for a checkup to determine the cause.

What is periodontitis?

Untreated gingivitis can advance to periodontitis, an infection of the tissues that hold your gums in place. Over time, plaque spreads and grows below the gum line, causing the gums to become swollen and red. The bacteria found in this plaque may irritate the gums, eventually breaking down the tissues and bone that support the teeth. The gums then separate from the teeth, forming spaces called pockets, which become infected. As the disease progresses, these pockets deepen, destroying more gum tissue and bone. A dentist can measure these pockets to determine the extent of the problem. Pockets measuring about 3 to 5 millimeters suggest gingivitis while pockets more than 5 millimeters indicate periodontitis. Eventually, teeth can become loose, fall out, or require removal.

Aggressive periodontitis can affect otherwise healthy young people. A condition called localized aggressive periodontitis is found in teenagers and young adults, affecting the first molars and incisors.

Medications That Cause Gingival Overgrowth

Seizure (or anticonvulsant) medications

Immunosuppressants (such as those used to treat psoriasis or prevent rejection of transplanted tissues)

Calcium channel blockers (often taken to treat high blood pressure)

If your child is taking any of these types of medications, talk to her pediatrician and dentist about any side effects that promote gingival overgrowth so that you can prevent any additional problems.

Saliva Test for Gum Disease

Researchers at Temple University have found that a simple color-changing oral strip can help detect gum disease more quickly and easily than traditional screening methods. The strip changes from white to yellow depending on levels of microbial sulfur compounds found in the saliva. A higher concentration of these compounds (and a darker shade of yellow) means a more serious case of gum disease. These strips aren't available for use by dentists yet, but be on the lookout for them and other new diagnostic tools to measure gum disease.

Even with little dental plaque or calculus, severe loss of alveolar bone occurs. Generalized aggressive periodontitis, on the other hand, may begin around puberty and involve the entire mouth. It is typically identified by inflammation of the gums and heavy accumulations of plaque and calculus.

What causes periodontal disease?

Dental plaque is the most common cause of gingivitis and periodontitis. More specifically, the bacteria in the plaque are the major offenders. Main causes of gum disease in children include genetics, poor oral hygiene, food frequently stuck in the gums, a deficiency of nutrients such as vitamin C, hormonal changes in puberty, ongoing teeth grinding, and certain medications, such as oral contraceptives and antidepressants.

Plaque is especially damaging if a child is in poor health or has a low resistance to disease. Some medical conditions increase the likelihood of a child developing periodontitis: diabetes, Down syndrome, or any disease (such as AIDS or kidney disease) or condition (such as taking antirejection drugs after an organ transplant) that reduces the amount of white blood cells in the body for extended periods and compromises the immune system.

Periodontal disease may be passed on to others when bacteria are passed from one person to another through saliva, including from parents to children and between couples. Genetics may also play a major role in the onset and severity of periodontal disease. Researchers found that up to 30 percent of the population may be genetically susceptible to developing severe periodontal disease. All of this adds up to the following advice: if one family member has periodontal disease, all family members should be screened for it by a dental professional.

Bleeding Gums: What to Do

If your child's gums bleed during brushing, she should try the following:

- Brush more often or more thoroughly, such as after every meal.
- Have her teeth professionally cleaned.
- Floss more often (but at least once each day) using proper flossing methods. Not flossing allows the bacteria to build up to dangerous levels.
- Consume less sugar, less often. Sugar helps plaque grow.
- Visit her dentist twice a year.
- Use a mouth rinse containing an antimicrobial agent, which removes excess bacteria.
- Use a high-quality electric toothbrush, which helps massage the gums.

Children with certain health conditions, like type 1 diabetes or Down syndrome, are at increased risk for developing periodontitis. Make sure you talk to your child's doctor about how your child's overall health may affect her chances of developing gum disease and how to prevent any further problems.

What is a periodontist?

If your child is having gum problems, his dentist might refer him to a periodontist, a specialist in diagnosing and treating gum disease. A periodontist is a dentist who has completed a postgraduate specialty program in periodontics after graduating from dental school.

Treating Gum Disease

Treatment depends on which stage of gum disease the child has and always involves oral hygiene and removal of bacterial plaque and hardened plaque, which is called tartar. Moderate to advanced gum disease usually requires a thorough cleaning of the teeth and teeth roots, called scaling and root planing and subgingival curettage. Scaling and root planing remove plaque and tartar from exposed teeth roots; subgingival curettage removes the surface of the inflamed layer of gum tissue. Both procedures are usually performed under local anesthesia to make them more comfortable.

Antibiotics are often prescribed with these procedures to stop the spread of infection and inflammation in the mouth and to treat abscesses. Antibiotics for treating gum disease may be taken in the form of medicated mouthwashes or antibiotic-containing gels or in fibers that are placed in gum pockets to slowly kill bacteria and help gums to heal.

A dentist or periodontist treating an advanced case of periodontitis may need to open and clean badly diseased gum pockets through surgery, then stitch the gums back into place to fit more snugly around the teeth. Gingival grafting may also be necessary, if gum tissue is so diseased that it cannot be sewn back together. In grafting, a dentist removes healthy gum tissue from another part of the mouth and stitches it in place of diseased tissue. The graft helps anchor the teeth, improving their appearance. In advanced gum disease with significant bone destruction and loosening of teeth, extractions may be necessary.

Early diagnosis is key to successful treatment of periodontal diseases. Children should have their gums examined as part of their routine dental visits. An advanced case of periodontal disease may also be an early sign of systemic disease. A general medical evaluation should be considered for children who have severe periodontitis, especially if the treatment does not appear to be working.

How can I help prevent my child's gum disease from returning?

Depending on the specific reason for your child's gum disease, you can help her make changes to reduce the likelihood of it returning after treatment. The most important preventive step against periodontal disease is to establish good oral health habits from the beginning.

- Mouth rinses are frequently used to help prevent gingivitis. Ask your child's dentist about appropriate medicated or prescription antibacterial mouthwashes that treat gum inflammation.
- Many medications can dry out the mouth or pose other threats to oral health. Be sure to tell your child's dentist about any medications she is taking.
- Teeth grinding can increase the risk of developing periodontal disease as well as causing cracked or chipped teeth. Dentists can make custom-fitted night bite guards to prevent teeth grinding while your child sleeps.
- Help your child maintain excellent nutrition and use vitamin supplements as recommended by her dentist or primary health care provider.
- Strongly discourage cigarettes and chewing tobacco, as they cause mouth irritation and are unhealthy for gums and teeth (and the rest of the body, too).

CHAPTER 14

Tooth Sensitivity and Pain

Children always seem to have pain somewhere. If it's not a headache, it's a bellyache. If it isn't the tummy, it might be the ear. Sometimes, it's a toothache. Pain around the teeth or jaws as a result of a dental condition will certainly demand our attention. Most toothaches are caused by a dental cavity, a cracked tooth, an exposed tooth root, or gum disease.

Some tooth pain isn't tooth pain at all, however. Inner ear or external ear infections and infection of the sinus cavities can cause tooth pain. Disorders of the jaw joint (temporomandibular joint) can also cause pain that is referred to as a toothache. The severity of a toothache can range from chronic and mild to sharp and excruciating. The pain may be aggravated by chewing or by cold or heat.

Dental Pain in Children

If your child complains of a toothache, ask him to point out the source of the ache. Is it a sharp pain, or just soreness around the tooth? A child may hide and keep quiet about a toothache or may exaggerate the pain. You'll need to investigate, to find out the facts of the matter.

In general, pain can be described as an unpleasant sensory and emotional experience. It is also a subjective experience, meaning that each person experiences pain differently. Many factors contribute to one's perception of pain, including biology, psychology, temperament, coping skills, cognitive development, context, previous experiences, culture, sensitivity, and parental anxiety.

Pain falls into one of two general categories: chronic or acute. Chronic pain is always there and continues for three months or longer. Acute pain is more brief but usually more intense than chronic pain. Acute dental pain in children is often associated with a tissue injury (such as a cut) or inflammation (as with a toothache or dental surgery). Regardless of the cause, pain should be taken seriously in children. Suffering can occur when the pain is overwhelming, nonstop, or out of control, or when the source of pain is unknown. Treating children's pain should be a priority for all health care and dental professionals as well as parents. Research shows that pain, especially unresolved pain, can have long-term consequences. For example, young children who undergo repeated painful procedures with inadequate pain control can develop fear and anxiety that later inhibits them from seeking necessary medical or dental care.

How is pain assessed in children?

Pain is often called the "fifth vital sign," and assessing pain is essential for managing it. Your child's doctor or dentist will take a medical history and perform a physical exam to determine the cause of the pain. The health care or dental professional will also use pain measurement tools, such as physiological (heart rate), behavioral, and self-report measures. The primary method of assessing pain in newborns, infants, children under 4, and children with developmental issues is to look for behavioral cues. Behaviors that may indicate pain include:

- Crying, whining, screaming, or other vocalizations
- Grimacing or similar facial expressions
- Withdrawing from caregivers
- Refusing to allow visual or physical inspection of suspected pain site

- Seeking comfort
- Agitated, irritable, tense, or angry mood
- Being inconsolable

Facial expression is the most reliable indicator of pain in infants and young children, but toddlers and preschoolers may be able to vocalize their pain, using words like "hurt" or "owie." Especially with younger children, caregivers need to describe to health care providers what's normal behavior for their child.

Children 4 to 8 years old may be able to indicate their level of pain on a face scale, a series of photographs or drawings of faces showing increased degrees of distress. Children 8 or older can verbally describe their pain, but they may need help answering questions about the severity or duration. A dentist will need to know not just that a child's mouth hurts but also

- how long it has been hurting
- what makes the pain better
- what makes the pain worse
- what the child was doing when the pain started (eating nuts, for example, or sleeping)

How do doctors and dentists figure out the cause of a child's dental pain?

Mouth pain such as a toothache is often a warning sign that something is wrong and needs to be evaluated. Your child's primary care provider can rule out sinus and ear problems. Consult your child's doctor first if pain is severe or accompanied by a fever, or if there is any drainage from the ears. A thorough oral examination by a dentist can help determine whether a toothache is coming from the mouth, a tooth, or the jaw. A minor toothache isn't an emergency but still warrants a call to the dentist for the next available appointment. A toothache that pain medicine can't even touch requires a call to the dental office's emergency number.

To identify the problem, a dentist will thoroughly assess your child's mouth for swelling, cuts, or sores. Next, the dentist may tap on your child's tooth to see if inflammation is present, rub the gum area near the end of the roots to check for sensitivity, and measure your child's gums to check the periodontal health of the area, including the "wiggliness" of teeth. The dentist might use a fiber optic light to check for cracks or fractures through the tooth. X-rays are usually taken from various angles to look for cavities, infections, or any other problems with the tooth anatomy.

What are dental causes of pain?

The most common cause of a toothache is a cavity. Cavities are holes in the two outer layers of a tooth (called the enamel and the dentin) caused when bacteria in the mouth convert simple sugars into acid. The acid softens and, along with saliva, dissolves the enamel and dentin, creating cavities. Small, shallow cavities may not cause pain or even be noticeable, but larger, deeper cavities can be very painful.

Another common cause of toothache is gum disease (see chapter 13). An early symptom of periodontal disease is gum bleeding without pain. Pain is often a symptom of more advanced gum disease, as the loss of bone around the teeth leads to the formation of deep gum pockets. Bacteria in these pockets cause gum infection, swelling, further bone destruction, and even more pain.

A toothache can also be caused by exposed tooth roots, a condition called recession. The roots are the lower two-thirds of teeth that are normally buried in bone. Bacterial toxins can dissolve this bone and cause the gum and the bone to recede, exposing the roots. The exposed roots can become extremely sensitive to cold, heat, and sour foods because they are no longer protected by healthy gum and bone. Early stages of root exposure can be treated with topical fluoride gels applied by the dentist or with special toothpastes made specifically for sensitive teeth. Dentists may also apply bonding agents to the exposed roots to seal the sensitive areas. If the root exposure causes injury to pulp tissue inside the tooth, additional treatment, such as a root canal procedure or tooth extraction, may be necessary.

Cracked tooth syndrome is tooth pain caused by a broken tooth, usually from chewing on or biting hard objects like hard candies, nuts, or ice. Biting on the cracked area can cause severe sharp pains. A dentist can usually detect the fracture by painting a special dye on the cracked tooth or shining a special light on it. Treatment for a cracked tooth usually involves covering the entire tooth with a crown.

> **Toothworms**
>
> In ancient times people believed that the stabbing pain of a toothache was caused by a toothworm that had drilled its way into the tooth. When the tooth pain was severe, the worm was supposed to be moving around, and as the aching stopped, the worm was apparently resting. The good news? No such worm exists. The bad news? Finding out what's causing tooth pain may be more complicated, because there are many possible causes.

In children, erupting teeth (growing out of the gums, or "cutting") can also be painful. When any tooth, especially molars, starts to come in, the surrounding gum can become inflamed and swollen. Dental pain can also stem from an impacted tooth, one that has failed to emerge into its proper position and remains under gum or bone. Impacted teeth cause pain when they put pressure on other teeth or bone or when they are inflamed or infected. This type of pain most often occurs with impacted wisdom teeth during the late teenage years.

Disorders of the temporomandibular joint or joints can cause pain, which usually occurs in or around the ears or lower jaw. Jaw disorders and pain are discussed in more detail in chapter 15.

Easing Toothache Pain

Toothaches can be hard on anyone, especially children, often leading to restless nights, nightmares, and loss of sleep for your child and you. If your child is scared and doesn't understand what is going on, he may even resist your efforts to bring him relief. However, it is important that you address his pain and try to figure out the cause as soon as possible.

Home remedies for toothaches might help manage the pain, but these are only short-term solutions until your child is able to see his dentist to determine the cause and find a more permanent solution. Here are few easy-to-use home remedies:

- Pay attention to foods. Avoid foods that are too hot, cold, hard, sticky, or sweet, which could further irritate the affected tooth.

- Although you shouldn't put ice directly on a sore tooth, you can use cool soft foods like cut-up potatoes, cucumbers, fruit, or berries instead. Tell your child to put the food on the tooth that is hurting and chew softly to soothe the pain. Also, you can use a cold pack on the outside of the mouth, remembering to put a towel or washcloth between the cold pack and the skin to avoid any skin irritation.

- Rinsing your child's mouth out with warm salt water can be helpful. You only need about 2 to 3 teaspoons of salt to a regular glass of warm water. If he refuses or doesn't like the salty taste, you can use regular water or apply a warm damp towel to his cheeks from the outside.

- Rub a little bit of garlic, or cashew oil on the affected tooth for their natural pain relief properties. Although clove oil works too, it can irritate the gums, so it should be carefully applied only to the tooth. Mint leaves or peppermint are also good for relieving pain.

Why Can't I Give Aspirin to My Child?

Children under age 17 should never be given aspirin, because it has been linked to Reye syndrome, a potentially deadly disease affecting the brain and the liver. The chances of developing Reye syndrome are small, but there is no need to take the risk when other pain relievers are available. Reye syndrome usually strikes children between the ages of 4 and 16—but rarely adults. Babies can get it, too, so if anyone in your house, or in a caregiver's home, takes baby aspirin to prevent heart problems, make sure it is kept in a locked cabinet.

What types of medications can relieve my child's tooth pain?

Some common over-the-counter medications may help. Children's acetaminophen (for example, Tylenol) is the pain and fever reliever of choice for many families. You should use only the type specifically identified for use by children (often in liquid or chewable form) and follow the directions for your child's age precisely; acetaminophen overdose is a serious matter.

Children's ibuprofen (for example Advil or Motrin) is another appropriate treatment for tooth pain if there's no bleeding or other contraindications, since ibuprofen can have a mild tendency to interfere with blood clotting. Again, use only the children's version and follow the directions exactly.

Children should never be given alcohol or aspirin as a pain medication, nor should they be given a medication packaged for adults. If your child's pain is severe or will not go away, consult your child's dentist or other health care professional right away.

How is pain managed during dental treatments?

Unfortunately, some dental problems and procedures can cause discomfort, but you and your child's dental team can take steps to limit, if not totally eliminate, your child's pain. Dealing with dental problems promptly can help prevent more serious problems, more painful procedures, and negative attitudes toward dental care that could last a lifetime.

The three keys to managing pain from dental procedures are:

- Controlling anxiety
- Communicating clearly about what to expect
- Preventing as much pain as possible

Effective pain management in children involves a combination of pharmacological, psychological, cognitive-behavioral, and physical treatments. Simple measures for dealing with a child in pain include:

- Reassurance, explanation, a calm environment, and gentle handling.
- Cognitive-behavioral techniques, such as teaching new behaviors and ways of thinking to cope with pain. These can include breathing techniques

Can I Use Numbing Gel on My Child's Teeth?

Topical pain reducers that have a numbing effect may be good short-term solutions for tooth-related pain. Manufacturers typically recommend that such numbing agents be used only with the advice of a medical professional. Adult products have a higher percentage of benzocaine than products designed for children and should therefore not be used in children. In fact, benzocaine is not recommended at all for very young children anymore. As with any medication, rare side effects can occur, so watch your child carefully after administering.

and helping children to focus away from the feared aspects of the dental procedure.

- Cold or hot packs.
- Oral analgesics and pain medication. Oral forms of pain medication are the most common drug therapy for children in pain. They are suitable for mild to moderate pain. Analgesic treatment should include proper dosing according to body weight, physiology, and the specific medical situation.
- Local anesthetics, or nerve blocks. Local anesthetics are used to stop the conduction of pain impulses through the nerves.
- Conscious sedation. These sedatives provide an amnesic effect, where the child does not remember any distress.

(For more information about the full range of anesthetics and sedation medication commonly used in dentistry, see chapter 19.)

My child's teeth seem sensitive. Is there anything I can do?

If your child complains of pain when eating ice cream or hot soup, sensitive teeth may be to blame. Sensitive teeth usually have a root cause.

For example, overenthusiastic vigorous brushing can lead to sensitive teeth. Many children do not know how to brush their teeth correctly. Ideally, the upper teeth should be brushed from top to bottom and the lower teeth from bottom to top, in small circular motions. Brushing our teeth horizontally, while applying a lot of force, wears down the outer surface of enamel. Sensitive teeth symptoms occur when the enamel wears thin, slightly exposing the dentin beneath, which tends to be very sensitive, especially to cold temperatures. To prevent sensitive teeth, teach your child to brush carefully and properly.

> *Honey, Onions, and Frogs*
>
> In the Middle Ages, honey was rubbed on aching teeth or a slice of onion was applied to the ear on the side of the aching tooth. The strangest theory? Spitting in a frog's mouth. If that didn't work, the frog was applied to the person's cheek on the side of the ailing tooth.

Another common cause of sensitive teeth in children is tooth decay. Tooth decay near the pulp causes sensitivity to hot or cold food as well as to sweets. Take your child to the dentist for treatment as soon as you realize she has a temperature-sensitive tooth, since this symptom may indicate a problem that needs immediate treatment. Some children continue to experience sensitive teeth after a filling, especially when the tooth decay is very close to the pulp. If this happens, talk to your child's dentist about options to lessen or eliminate the pain.

Does special toothpaste for sensitive teeth really work?

Many kinds of toothpaste for sensitive teeth can help prevent sensitivity when eating or drinking hot or cold food or beverages. Toothpaste designed for sensitive teeth can be a solution to a long-term but harmless sensitivity or just a stopgap solution to a more serious problem, such as a cavity near the pulp. Rather than waiting for this problem to get worse, take your child to the dentist and get the condition diagnosed and treated as soon as possible.

CHAPTER 15

Conditions of the Mouth, Tongue, and Jaw

Good oral health involves more than just the teeth and gums. The tongue, lips, cheeks, and jaw are all important to children's health, including their ability to eat nutritious foods. Taking care of the whole mouth will help keep your child eating well and feeling well.

Dry Mouth

Saliva has many important jobs: to moisten and cleanse our mouths, to help digest food, and to control bacteria and fungi in the mouth, preventing infections. When we don't produce enough saliva, our mouth gets dry and uncomfortable. In clinical terms, dry mouth is referred to as xerostomia.

Saliva is produced by different glands located throughout the mouth. Beneath the tongue is the area known as the floor of the mouth, where a thin strip of tissues, called the lingual frenulum (or frenum), connects the floor of the mouth to the tongue. Near the attachment of the frenulum to the mouth floor are the tiny openings (ducts) of the two submandibular salivary glands. These ducts are called the submandibular ducts, or Wharton's ducts. The ducts of the two sublingual salivary glands are located on either side of the Wharton's ducts. In addition, there are two large salivary glands, known as the parotid glands. The parotid glands are located

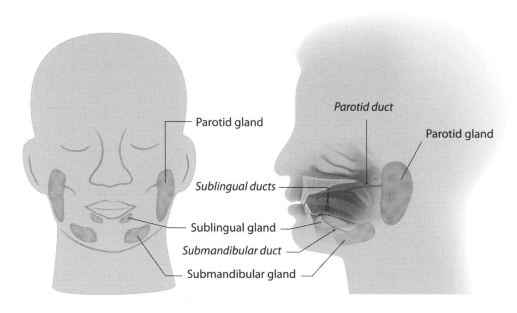

The salivary glands and ducts. Courtesy of hkann / Shutterstock.com

along the sides of the jaw, just below and in front of the ears, between the masseter muscle (which helps us chew) and the skin. These glands empty through tiny holes called Stenson's ducts, which appear as small bumps on the insides of our cheeks, near the maxillary (upper) second molars. If any of these glands fails to make enough saliva, a person gets dry mouth.

Common symptoms of dry mouth include:

- A sticky, dry feeling in the mouth
- Frequent thirst
- Sores in the mouth
- Sores or split skin at the corners of the mouth
- Cracked lips
- A dry feeling in the throat
- A burning or tingling sensation in the mouth and especially on the tongue

- A dry, red, raw tongue
- Problems speaking or tasting, chewing, and swallowing
- Hoarseness
- Dry nasal passages
- Sore throat
- Bad breath

What causes dry mouth?

There are several causes of dry mouth, including:

- *Medications.* Many prescription and nonprescription drugs, including drugs used to treat depression, anxiety, pain, allergies, colds, acne, epilepsy, high blood pressure, diarrhea, nausea, or asthma can cause dry mouth.
- *Diseases and infections.* Dry mouth can be a side effect of certain medical conditions, including Sjogren syndrome, HIV/AIDS, diabetes, anemia, cystic fibrosis, rheumatoid arthritis, high blood pressure, stroke, or cancer.
- *Nerve damage.* Injury or surgery to the head and neck area in which there is nerve damage can result in dry mouth.
- *Tobacco use.* Smoking or chewing tobacco affects saliva production and aggravates dry mouth.
- *Mouth breathing.* Breathing with your mouth open can also contribute to the problem.

A dry sticky mouth in children may also be a sign of dehydration. Dehydration can be caused by not drinking enough fluids, excessive sweating after physical activity, or an illness with fever, diarrhea, or vomiting. When your child has a fever, more water evaporates from his body as his temperature increases. If your child cannot replace the lost fluids, he may become dehydrated. Other signs of dehydration include few or no tears when crying, eyes that look sunken, lack of urine, dry cool skin, lethargy or fatigue, irritability, or dizziness.

The goal of treating dehydration is to restore the normal levels of body fluids by replacing fluids lost. Children who are dehydrated should drink water at first, but they may need additional fluids containing electrolytes, sold at grocery stores and pharmacies. Electrolytes help the body absorb the right combination of sugar and salts. If you suspect that your child is dehydrated and he shows no improvement, or the dehydration is worsening, you need to contact your child's doctor immediately to prevent serious complications.

Why is dry mouth a problem and how is it treated?

Dry mouth causes the aggravating symptoms mentioned above, and it also increases your child's risk of gingivitis (gum disease), tooth decay, and mouth infections, such as thrush. Plus, having a dry mouth can be just plain uncomfortable.

To prevent dry mouth, your child should drink plenty of fluids during exercise. If your child has fever, diarrhea, or vomiting, make sure she consumes more liquids than she is losing. This may be difficult if she is not feeling well, but it is important to keep offering liquids to her.

If you think your child's dry mouth is caused by medications she is taking, talk to her doctor, who might adjust the dose or switch your child to a different drug that doesn't cause dry mouth. In addition, her doctor might prescribe an oral rinse to restore mouth moisture. If that doesn't help, a medication that stimulates saliva production, called pilocarpine (Salagen), may be prescribed.

Other steps you can take that may help improve saliva flow:

- Encourage your child to suck on sugar-free candy or chew sugar-free gum.
- Make sure she drinks plenty of water to help keep her mouth moist.

Chapped Lips

We all know that chapped lips hurt. When your child licks her lips, she is momentarily applying moisture, but when it evaporates, her lips will feel drier than before. Saliva contains digestive enzymes that don't do sore lips any good. Licking chapped lips can lead to something called lip-licker's dermatitis, which is red, irritated skin around the mouth. To prevent chapped lips in your child, keep the air in your home moist with a humidifier, buy beeswax-based lip balm for your child to wear, and protect her lips when she is out in the sun, cold, or wind.

- Encourage your child to breathe through her nose, not her mouth, as much as possible.
- Use a room vaporizer to add moisture to bedroom air.

Other Common Mouth Conditions

What is a mouth ulcer?

A mouth ulcer is probably the most common of all oral diseases. It is a white lesion or open sore that can appear anywhere in the mouth. It most often appears as a result of an injury.

Causes of ulcers include biting lips or tongue, often after dental work, when the mouth is still numb from a local anesthetic. Hot foods, like pizza, can burn the soft tissues of the mouth, resulting in an ulcer. Sometimes acidic foods, like many fruits, lemon juice, vinegar, and tomatoes, can cause painful white ulcers. Mouth ulcers usually disappear within two to three weeks but may persist for longer.

My child tends to suck his lips. Is this bad?

Lip sucking involves repeatedly holding the lower lip against the upper front teeth. Some children who suck their lip also suck their thumb. Both habits can result in an overbite and other structural problems. In addition, lip sucking often leads to red and irritated skin around the mouth, which can be particularly painful in the winter. Because of the potential for discomfort and long-term dental problems, lip sucking should be treated like thumb sucking and consistently discouraged.

What is a canker sore?

Also called aphthous ulcers, canker sores are fairly common painful white ulcers that vary in size. They may appear singly, or in groups, and often recur. No one is sure of the exact cause. They may be brought on by stress or triggered by sodium lauryl sulfate, an ingredient found in toothpaste. They usually last for ten to fourteen days and are treated by using bland mouthwashes and applying topical anesthetics and protective ointments.

What's the difference between a cold sore and canker sore?

Cold sores and canker sores are often confused with each other, but they are not the same. Cold sores are often called fever blisters or herpes simplex type 1. Unlike canker sores, cold sores are usually caused by a virus that can pass from person to person. If your child has a sore and you're wondering if it's of the cold or canker variety, just look at where it's located. Cold sores show up outside the mouth, around the lips, chin, or nostrils, while canker sores are always found inside the mouth.

Can children get mouth cysts?

A cyst is an abnormal swelling, usually small, that contains a clear fluid. It is painless unless it becomes infected. The most common types of mouth cysts in children are:

• *Mucoceles.* These small, ball-shaped, painless swellings are caused by injury to the small salivary glands and are usually located on the lip or palate. They can burst spontaneously, disappear, and recur.

• *Eruption cysts.* These cysts are swellings of the gum over baby or permanent teeth before eruption. They are sometimes filled with blood, giving them a bluish color. When the tooth erupts into the mouth, they usually rupture (burst) and disappear.

• *Dentigerous cysts.* The most common cyst in the jaws of children, a dentigerous cyst forms around the crown of a permanent tooth before it erupts. It is usually painless and is generally discovered on x-ray. The eruption of a tooth may be delayed by such a cyst.

• *Radicular cysts.* These cysts form around the root of a permanent tooth in which the nerves and blood vessels have died. Baby teeth do not usually form this type of cyst. They are usually painless and can be treated by root canal.

Why are the corners of my son's mouth crusting and cracking?

Angular cheilitis (often called just cheilitis) is a fairly common skin problem at the junction of lip and facial skin, usually at the corner of the mouth. Cheilitis brings inflammation, burning, redness, and ulceration or cracks around the skin on the lip. The affected area is often itchy and painful. In more advanced cases, the cracks may bleed when the mouth is opened. These open lesions may form a crust as they start to heal, or they may become infected. Eating and speaking can be uncomfortable—and can make the problem worse.

Angular cheilitis occurs for many reasons. It can be caused by a fungal, or yeast, infection (candidiasis), a bacterial (staphylococcal) infection, or a viral infection. People taking a medication called isotretinoin to treat acne are more vulnerable to cheilitis. It may also be caused by iron or various B vitamin deficiencies, constant lip licking or biting, thumb sucking, bottle feeding, sucking on pacifiers, loss of teeth, sun exposure, wind and cold air exposure, or a weakened immune system. Having certain skin conditions, such as atopic or seborrheic dermatitis, may make a person more vulnerable to cheilitis. Skin sensitivities to toothpastes and cosmetics can also cause this lip problem. Some foods or drinks, such as citrus, can make the problem worse.

Depending on the cause, cheilitis can be treated or prevented in many ways. For example, your child should avoid irritating his lips by constant lip licking or biting. Thumb sucking or using a pacifier should also be stopped if signs of cheilitis appear. Using a moisturizing lip balm with UV protection when outside is also helpful. If a certain cosmetic or toothpaste is causing irritation, your child should stop using it.

Cheilitis caused by a fungal or bacterial infection can be treated with topical antifungal or antibacterial medicated gels applied to the affected areas. If a deficiency in the B vitamins is detected, your child could take supplements or focus on eating more foods that provide the B vitamins. Consult your health care provider about treatments for cheilitis.

Is there anything I can do to make eating less painful for my daughter while the cut in her mouth heals?

A lesion on the inside of the mouth can be painful, and trying to eat can be excruciating. As a caregiver, you'll want to look for ways to minimize discomfort and maximize the nutritional value of every bite your child gets down. A diet of enriched milkshakes may not be a good idea long term, but if it keeps your child satisfied and healthy for a few days, then it's the perfect fuel. You can help her in other ways as well:

> *Mouth Sores—When to Call a Health Care Provider*
>
> If your child has a mouth sore and any of these situations arise, call his health care provider:
>
> - Pain becomes severe.
> - The sore does not begin to heal within a week.
> - The area looks infected (increasing pain, redness, or swelling after 48 hours).
> - Your child develops a fever.
> - He has difficulty drinking or swallowing.

- Encourage your child to drink her favorite fluids to prevent dehydration. Cold drinks, milkshakes, and Popsicles are especially good.
- Offer a soft diet rather than foods that need a lot of chewing.
- Make sure she avoids salty or citrus foods, which might sting.
- Rinse the wound with warm water immediately after meals.

My son is a mouth breather. How will this affect his long-term health?

Mouth breathing simply refers to inhaling and exhaling through the mouth. A healthy person normally breathes through the nose while resting or doing light exercise, and breathes through both the nose and mouth during vigorous aerobic exercise. Mouth breathing may not sound like a problem, but it can have devastating effects on general health and growth. Many seemingly unrelated but serious conditions are linked to mouth breathing, such as chronic allergies, tonsil hypertrophy, nasal polyps, deviated nasal septum, constricted upper airways, and a backward positioned lower jaw caused by thumb sucking, excessive pacifier use, or insufficient sucking as an infant.

One of the more serious complications of mouth breathing is that many children are misdiagnosed with attention deficit disorder (ADD) and hyperactivity. Children who mouth breathe typically do not sleep well, so they are tired during the day and often unable to concentrate in school, resulting in poor performance. In addition, mouth breathing can cause low oxygen levels in the bloodstream, which can lead to high blood pressure, heart problems, sleep apnea, and other serious medical issues.

The common symptoms of mouth breathing include:

- Long, narrow face or other issues with facial structure development
- Difficulty breathing through the nose
- Delayed physical growth
- Dry lips
- Dark circles under eyes
- Excessive creases between lower lip and chin
- Allergies
- Smaller jaws with crowded teeth
- Swollen tonsils
- Bad breath
- High rate of tooth decay

If it is not properly treated, mouth breathing can lead to many serious problems, including the following.

COMPROMISED AIRWAY

Mouth breathing can cause a compromised airway. Airway problems can also be caused by the lower jaw, along with the tongue, being positioned too far back, constricting the upper airway. Chronic allergies can lead to enlarged tonsils and adenoids, which may be the common cause for many cases of mouth breathing, although mouth breathing in itself will increase tonsil size, thus constricting the airway to such an extent that breathing normally through the nose becomes nearly impossible.

OBSTRUCTIVE SLEEP APNEA

If a compromised airway from mouth breathing isn't corrected, it can lead to snoring and eventually obstructive sleep apnea (OSA). In children, OSA symptoms can include bed-wetting, poor quality of sleep, obesity, and behavioral symptoms resembling ADHD. In adults, OSA is a silent killer. Most snorers are not aware that they may be suffering from OSA. Over time, snoring due to OSA increases the risk for cardiovascular disease, stroke, obesity, high blood pressure, and diabetes.

> *Is It Sleep Apnea?*
>
> The BEARS acronym stands for symptoms that could point to sleep apnea:
>
> Bedtime problems, such as nightmares
> Excessive daytime sleepiness
> Awakenings at night
> Regularity and duration of sleep affected
> Snoring

ALTERED HEAD AND NECK POSTURE

Mouth breathing can also cause posture problems. The unnatural process of regularly breathing through the mouth, which makes children look like they are gasping for air, leads to a forward head posture. This posture puts stress on the upper back and neck muscles, which over time can lead to permanent posture changes, such as abnormal curvatures in the spine and shoulders.

CAVITIES AND GUM DISEASE

Mouth breathing changes the bacterial flora in the mouth, which can lead to cavities and gum disease.

WEAKENED IMMUNE SYSTEM AND POOR HEALTH

Nasal breathing helps regulate normal blood circulation. It also filters, warms, and moisturizes the air breathed in. The lack of oxygen in mouth breathers, who usually snore at night and struggle for air, weakens the immune system, disrupts deep sleep cycles, and interferes with growth hormone production.

POOR PERFORMANCE

The lack of oxygen and its effects on growth hormones increase the tendency for mouth-breathing children to be overweight and tired, which causes lack of concentration and poor performance in school and in athletics. Additionally, being tired and irritable can lead to behavior problems.

How is mouth breathing treated?

Mouth breathing in children should be addressed as soon as possible by first talking with your child's pediatrician or dentist, or an ear-nose-throat (ENT) specialist, who is experienced in treating children with this condition. Mouth breathing in children is often caused by enlarged adenoids, underdeveloped nasal passages, or nasal blockages. Regardless of the cause, the following steps are frequently recommended to help clear nasal passages, allowing your child to breathe better:

• *Allergy screening.* If you suspect an allergy, have your child screened by an allergist. Depending on the results, eliminate potential allergens from your home, such as pollen, dust, mold, animal dander, or chemicals. If your child is allergic to certain foods, such as dairy, preservatives, dyes, artificial sweeteners, or other additives, eliminate these as well. Some children may also have a sensitivity or intolerance to yeasts or gluten. In any case, your allergist can help you develop an appropriate diet for your child.

• *Natural remedies.* Many natural remedies are thought to address allergies, such as neti pots, saline, and steam. Craniosacral, osteopathic, or massage therapies can also help to increase circulation of blood, lymph, and cerebrospinal fluids, lessening allergies.

> *The World's Longest Tongue*
>
> Guinness World Record holder Stephen Taylor of the United Kingdom has a tongue that extends 3.86 inches from tip to top lip.

Common Tongue Conditions

The tongue is mainly composed of muscles and is covered with a mucus membrane. The ventral surface, or underside, of the tongue, is smooth and is not involved in the sense of taste. The dorsal, or top, surface of the tongue is what you can see most clearly when you look in the mirror. It is covered with hairlike projections called filiform papillae. Between the papillae are the taste buds. The tongue has two primary functions—to help us chew and swallow by moving food around and to help us form words.

Could my daughter's taste buds be inflamed?

As you probably remember from grade school, there are five prime elements of taste: salty, sour, bitter, sweet, and savory. The main function of the taste buds is to taste or savor the foods we eat, differentiate the tastes, and send this information to the brain.

Taste buds may become inflamed for several reasons:

- Hot, spicy, or salty foods
- Acidic foods, including lemons, limes, grapefruit, and some sauces
- Overcooked foods, which are physically hot
- Exposure to toxins like tobacco smoke and insecticides
- Certain herbs and supplements
- Stomach infection or allergy
- A cut on the taste bud
- Mouth ulcers or tongue ulcers
- A yeast (thrush) infection
- Certain mineral or vitamin deficiencies
- Endocrine disorders, such as hypothyroidism and diabetes
- Dental problems
- Surgery affecting the mouth or throat

Inflammation of the taste buds can affect how food tastes or cause soreness, irritation, and swelling. Inflamed taste buds due to a cut can be cured by applying glycerin on the affected area. An injury caused by a burn will feel better and heal more quickly if your child sucks on ice chips and eats soft, cold foods.

Should I be concerned about changes in my son's tongue color?

Your child's tongue color can reflect dietary deficiencies or other problems. For example, iron deficiency anemia or a vitamin B12 deficiency may make the tongue look pale and smooth. The first sign of scarlet fever may be a change from the tongue's normal color to a strawberry, and then raspberry, color. A constant strawberry-red tongue in a young child may also be a sign of Kawasaki disease, an autoimmune disease. A smooth, red tongue and painful mouth may indicate a lack of niacin in the diet.

My daughter has these weird patches on her tongue that seem to come and go. What are they?

The most common concern related to children's tongues is called a geographic tongue, where lighter colored patches resembling a map spread out on the top surface. The patches are areas of missing papillae, and they are smooth and red, often with slightly raised borders. The appearance of the tongue changes from day to day because the lesions often heal in one area and then move (migrate) to a different part of the tongue. Geographic tongue is also known as benign migratory glossitis.

Although geographic tongue may look alarming, it isn't usually associated with any serious health problems. In some people, geographic tongue causes discomfort and increased sensitivity to certain foods. Common aggravators include pineapple, walnuts, eggplant, and spicy foods. People who have psoriasis, allergies, eczema, or asthma are more likely to have geographic tongue. It occurs in around 2 percent of people of all ages, sexes, and races, affecting females three times more than males and more often appearing in adults than in children.

The condition is benign and does not require treatment, although some people report an improvement in the condition when they take a multivitamin daily, and others claim to have success with vitamin B or zinc supplementation. Before adding nutritional supplements to your child's diet, consult with her health care provider. Using a tongue brush or tongue scraper twice a day may help. Let your older children know that alcohol and smoking can also be triggers.

How do I know if my son has thrush on his tongue?

Thrush on the tongue looks like a coat of white spots. It is caused by the *Candida* fungus, a type of yeast. Thrush in children often comes on after the child completes a round of antibiotics or has an illness. It tends to be painful, because there are lesions under the white coating. If the coating is scraped in some way, bleeding may begin. Since it is a yeast infection, it can also spread to the throat or other areas of the body. If you aren't sure whether your child has thrush, check in with his dentist or pediatrician. If thrush is found, antifungal medications can be prescribed, which should clear up the infection in about 10 to 14 days.

My daughter ate something and now her tongue is swelling. What should I do?

Swelling of the tongue must always be taken seriously and addressed right away. The swelling can spread quickly (sometimes within minutes), eventually obstructing the airway and making breathing difficult or even impossible.

Different situations can trigger swelling of the tongue. With food allergies, swelling is usually accompanied by other symptoms, such as itching, hives, wheezing, or vomiting. Allergies to medications (including over-the-counter medications) also cause similar symptoms, including swelling. Other causes for swelling of the tongue include infections, trauma, or insect bites or stings. Ask relatives on both sides of your child's family if they ever had problems with severe allergies or sudden swelling. Sometimes these conditions can be hereditary, and this information can let you know what to watch for in your child.

The best way to prevent tongue swelling from happening again is to figure out the cause and avoid it. Review all foods, drinks, candies, and medications taken within a few hours before the swelling started. Allergies to foods or medicines are treated by stopping the food or medication completely and labeling your child's medical record clearly to make sure she never receives the culprit product again. Children should also be aware if they are allergic to insect bites or stings as well so they can notify an adult immediately if they encounter an issue, especially if you are not with them.

Regardless of the reason for the swelling or its severity, any children with a history of swelling, especially of the tongue or mouth area, should see their doctor or allergist about allergy testing and a prescription for an epinephrine self-injector pen (often called an EpiPen) and be taught how to use it correctly. Epinephrine helps control the swelling to give your child time to get to the doctor or hospital to prevent any breathing difficulties or other major problems. Sometimes you will need to purchase several EpiPens so that your child can keep one at school, one at the babysitter's, and one in the home of each friend and family member she visits often just in case any reaction or swelling occurs.

> *Protect against Summer Stings*
>
> Remind your child to never leave opened cans of soda or other sweetened drinks outside. Bees and other stinging insects can hide inside the can and then sting an unsuspecting drinker. Using a straw or a cup with a lid can also protect against such stings. Wasps, yellow jackets, bumblebees, and hornets can sting repeatedly (unlike honeybees), since their stingers do not come off in the skin. Bee stings can quickly cause a severe, even fatal, reaction if not immediately addressed.

Why does my child chew his tongue?

Tongue chewing may be one of the most common unrecognized and undocumented habits in children and adults, affecting millions of people. Medical journals and the Internet carry an abundance of information about various oral habits and movement disorders; however, tongue chewing is rarely discussed, studied, or documented. Most tongue chewers start the habit in early childhood, between 5 months and 5 years old, though tongue chewing can begin at any age, including earlier than 5 months or in teenagers and adults.

It may have started with thumb sucking, teething, or tongue thrusting, or as a tension reducer that evolved into a repetitive habitual behavior.

Sometimes symptoms start from an emotional or physical trauma. Some people who chew their tongues are unaware that they are doing it, while for others, it is an annoying and embarrassing chronic habit.

In mild cases, the person may only occasionally bite lightly on one or both sides of the tongue and may be completely unaware of doing it. In more severe cases, the tongue chewing is intense and includes a forward or lateral (side-to-side) tongue thrust. Tongue chewing movements may also include squirming or twisting. Some people also contort the jaw, cause clicking and popping in the temporomandibular joint. The tongue may be dry, tender, and sore, and it may have teeth marks on both sides or on just one side. Some people also make noises, including clicking or humming. Tongue chewing shares characteristics with other repetitive behavior and movement and tic disorders, such as nail biting, thumb sucking, bruxism (teeth grinding), and trichotillomania (hair pulling).

> **Tongue Chewing in Infancy**
>
> Some babies start tongue chewing when teeth are emerging. If your baby has a sore tongue from chewing, do not put a numbing agent on her tongue. If the pain is numbed, she may bite harder, causing even more damage.

The chewing often begins unconsciously and can be suppressed for only minutes at a time. Once there is a distraction from the intention not to chew, the chewing begins again. Yet many people also have periods when they do not chew—for days or even years, and some are able to avoid doing it in public. Symptoms are often worse when the person is stressed, bored, distracted, or excited. Chewing sometimes subsides when the person is lying down and may not be present during sleep. There is a pacifying, pleasurable aspect to chewing.

If your child chews his tongue, schedule a dental visit to rule out any structural problems. You may also want to schedule a visit with his pediatrician for an iron-level

> **What Is Orofacial Myofunctional Therapy?**
>
> For children and teens with problems related to oral and facial muscles, an orofacial myofunctional therapist may help correct longstanding problems. Orofacial therapy is a program used to correct the improper function of the tongue and facial muscles used at rest, for chewing, and for swallowing. You can find a qualified therapist in your area by visiting the International Association of Orofacial Myology directory page on www.iaom.com.

screening, because anemia can sometimes cause tongue swelling, which can increase the likelihood of tongue chewing. If everything looks normal, an orofacial myofunctional therapist can help retrain your child's muscles.

What does it mean when a child is tongue tied?

The expression "tongue tied" generally makes us think of someone who is too nervous or excited to speak. The expression comes from a common physical condition called ankyloglossia, where the use of the tongue is limited by a problem with the lingual frenulum, the cord of tissue that basically "ties" the tongue to the floor of the mouth.

The job of the frenulum is simple—it guides the development of the mouth and then the position of incoming teeth, thinning out as children grow. The frenulum is usually fairly elastic, so it does not interfere with the movements of the tongue in sucking, eating, clearing food off the teeth before swallowing, and, of course, speech.

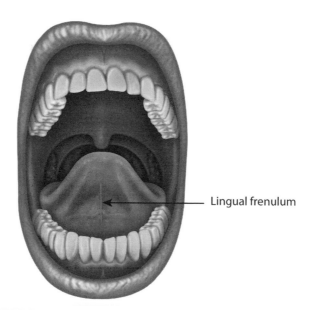

Lingual frenulum

The lingual frenulum. If the frenulum is too tight, it can lead to a condition called ankyloglossia, often referred to as being tongue tied. © Can Stock Photo Inc. / alexilus

In some children, the frenulum either doesn't thin out or is especially tight, which can cause tongue mobility problems. When it is short, thick, tight, or broad, the frenulum can restrict feeding and speech. It can also cause problems when it extends too far across the floor of the mouth to finish at the base of the teeth. Being tongue tied with a too tight frenulum can require a procedure called a lingual frenectomy, the surgical removal of the frenulum, sometimes called "clipping the tongue." The procedure is quick and easy to do on newborns, but can be more complicated as children get older. After the procedure, the tongue can usually be completely extended and becomes fully mobile.

A frenulum can also be found underneath the center of the upper lip. If this frenulum is attached too far down the gum, it can cause the gums to recede and create gaps between the front teeth. The surgical removal of this tissue, called a labial frenectomy, is a simple procedure that is often performed in a doctor's or dentist's office. Patients rarely experience any complications from the surgery, and it can often correct or prevent problems related to excess tissue.

All tongue ties do not look alike. They can be thin and membranous, thick and white, short, long or wide, extending from the margin of the tongue all the way to the lower front teeth, or so short and tight that they make a web connecting the tongue to the floor of the mouth. Tongue tie often runs in families. Some relatives may have only mild effects or no apparent symptoms, while others have a severe case that affects the structure and function of their mouths. If your child has tongue tie, you may notice similarities to other relatives with the condition, especially when your child is older. Similarities in lips and tongue, habits of speech, and nose and face shapes are common.

Some children who have other congenital conditions that affect the structure of the mouth, such as cleft lip or palate, or conditions such as severe hearing loss or cerebral palsy, also have tongue tie. More boys have tongue tie than girls.

Different professions use their own means and different methods of identifying and assessing tongue tie, such as by

- measuring "free tongue" and the height to which the tongue can be lifted
- looking at the appearance of the margin of the tongue and whether an indentation is present
- assessing the function of the tongue and the child's ability to protrude or elevate the tongue
- discussing whether any problems were experienced with breastfeeding
- identifying any speech problems

Early intervention is ideal, so your child does not form habits or suffer the negative effects of messy or slow eating, "funny-looking" teeth, or speech problems. Fewer bad habits will make it easier to correct the difficulties poor tongue mobility has caused. Once a tongue tie has been diagnosed, the next step is usually to remove the frenulum. Any remaining problems can then be treated, nearly always successfully.

What type of treatment is most appropriate? That depends on the problems the child is experiencing. A lactation consultant can help with correcting poor sucking, which will improve breastfeeding. A speech-language pathologist can help with speech and language problems. A dentist or orthodontist can help with crooked or decayed teeth and infected gums. The sooner the structural problem is corrected, the better.

Common Jaw Conditions

Many jaw problems develop at an early age. Adult teeth may grow in wrong, or the child's jaw may have been malformed since birth. Some problems, such as temporomandibular joint (TMJ) disorders or teeth grinding, often appear in childhood but don't become a problem until adulthood. Jaw issues should be identified as early as possible by a doctor or a dentist and fixed before they get worse.

Tooth alignment. Permanent teeth in the back of the mouth can sometimes become lodged in the jaw as they are coming in, leading to pain and jaw malformation. Poor tooth alignment is corrected by a combination of surgery and orthodontics. Basically, a hole is drilled into the jaw and braces are used to slowly coax the lodged tooth out of the hole.

Jaw malformation. Malformation of the jaw, as the name indicates, is a condition in which the jaw does not develop properly, causing pain, especially when eating. Overbites and underbites are common jaw malformations. Other malformations are caused by the jaw attempting to compensate for overcrowding or for baby teeth that have become lodged in the bone. Malformations are fixed by orthodontics or surgery.

Teeth grinding. Children can develop the habit of clenching or grinding their teeth, called bruxism. Usually the habit is a subconscious one, often occurring during sleep. Teeth grinding can indicate a TMJ disorder, but it is usually a habit developed out of stress. Bruxism is common among children, particularly during the years when permanent teeth are coming in, and most will outgrow it. If not, or if pain continues, talk to your child's dentist.

What are TMJ disorders?

TMJ disorders include various conditions related to the temporomandibular joint, the joint that connects the lower jaw to the skull. You can actually feel this joint by placing your fingers directly in front of your ears and opening your mouth. The TMJ is important because it helps with chewing, swallowing, and speech.

TMJ disorders can affect children of any age, but they are more common during the teenage years, among girls, and in people who have other dental problems (like a bad bite), joint problems (like arthritis), muscle problems, or a history of trauma to the jaw or face. Although it is often not clear what causes TMJ disorders, jaw clenching or teeth grinding can increase the chance of developing a problem. Constant grinding and clenching can overwork the joint or move it out of place, affecting the bite. Most people don't even realize that they're clenching, grinding, or tightening their jaws, especially because many do it while they sleep or when stressed. However, a dentist can easily recognize TMJ issues, which makes regular dental appointments even more important. If your child's dentist suspects a TMJ problem, she might recommend additional x-rays, CT scans, or an MRI to assess the severity and confirm a diagnosis. The earlier a TMJ disorder is diagnosed and treated, the better.

Many symptoms can indicate a problem with the TM joint. Some of the most common are

- pain or soreness around the teeth or in the facial muscles, jaw joints, near the ears, or sometimes in the neck and shoulders
- jaw pain when talking, chewing, biting, or yawning
- popping, clicking, or grating sounds when opening or closing the mouth
- difficulty or stiffness when opening or closing the mouth, sometimes with jaw locking
- headaches or earaches without another cause

If your child has symptoms of a TMJ disorder, let her dentist know.

How are TMJ disorders treated?

For some children with TMJ disorders, treatment can be relatively simple and involve only self-care. Your child might be told to rest his jaw for a few days whenever it becomes tender. Offer him soft foods and make sure he avoids hard or chewy foods that might strain his jaw muscles. Apply moist heat to the side of the face to help relax his jaw muscles.

Monitor your child's stress and anxiety levels. Lots of people develop TMJ disorders or joint pain as they get older after years of unconsciously and repeatedly grinding their teeth or clenching the jaw due to stress. It is important that your child learn to control these habits early on. Teach him to notice these stress-related behaviors so that he can consciously stop them as soon as they start to happen. Regular exercise can also help release nervous energy in children, preventing stress overloads.

When self-care is not enough, physical therapy by a trained professional often helps to reduce jaw pain. This therapy uses stretching and strengthening jaw exercises, deep heat therapies, and biofeedback.

Depending on the specific diagnosis, further treatment might be necessary. If pain is caused by clenching the jaw or grinding the teeth, the dentist may fit your child with a bite guard to wear at night or during stressful periods when teeth grinding or jaw clenching are likely. Medication might be prescribed to help relieve the pain or relax the muscles, allowing for easier jaw movement. If a problem with your child's bite is contributing to the TMJ disorder, his dentist might recommend braces or other dental work to correct it and lessen the stress on the jaw. Although most children do not require surgery, some children with severe TMJ problems will need it to eliminate the pain better and faster. Some TMJ surgeries include lubricating the joint to reduce inflammation or pain, removing cartilage fragments or scar tissue, reshaping or replacing the joint, or correcting jaw misalignment.

What causes an overbite?

Overbites are common in children and often genetic. Thumb sucking, finger sucking, or other habits that force the upper teeth out over the lower teeth can worsen an existing overbite or even cause one. Sometimes breathing disorders cause overbite. The first and best treatment for many children is to stop thumb sucking or other bad habits that can make their overbite more severe.

For years, overbites weren't treated until the children were old enough for braces. The problems with waiting this long, however, are that overbites can make chewing difficult, increase the child's risk for dental trauma, and be a source of teasing in school. These days, overbites are often treated effectively in young children. An overbite is normally a difference in the way the jaw bones are aligned, with the lower jaw back too far. Orthopedic appliances can help bring the lower jaw forward.

There are several to choose from depending on the needs of your child. These appliances work by guiding the jaws into alignment during their natural growth process, which is the main reason orthopedic appliances work much better in children than they do in adults, whose jaws are no longer growing. The best ages are between about 7 and 14. By the time your child is 16, an untreated overbite will already be much more difficult to correct.

Examine your child's teeth. If there is any question whether he has an overbite, seek out her dentist's opinion. It is crucial to evaluate children as young as 5 years old for developing bite problems. Untreated developmental problems can lead to headaches, ear pain, jaw pain, facial pain, sinus congestion, and neck problems.

What is an underbite?

Ideally, when you close your upper and lower jaws, the upper teeth are located just ahead of the lower teeth. If instead your lower teeth are located ahead of your upper teeth, you have an underbite. Between 5 and 10 percent of the general population have underbites. The frequency is higher among people who are Asian.

Underbites in children are common and often resolve on their own as more permanent teeth come in. An underbite can be either skeletal or dental. Skeletal underbite occurs when the lower jaw is too far forward compared with the upper jaw. This condition may be hereditary or due to long-term behaviors like thumb sucking. Dental underbite is usually caused by a crossbite. Crossbite occurs when one or more of the lower teeth are located outside the upper teeth when the two jaws are in occlusion. This can occur at the front of the mouth or the sides. When it occurs at the front, it creates a dental underbite. The tooth or teeth are slightly forwardly placed, not the entire lower jaw.

Your child may simply appear to have an underbite because all his teeth haven't fully erupted yet. Make an appointment for him with an orthodontist, who can tell whether your child has a true underbite. If he does, then appropriate treatment should be started. Uncorrected, an underbite can lead to TMJ disorders. Many years of living with an underbite can cause the teeth to wear down prematurely or unevenly.

I had to have surgery for my underbite. Is that the only treatment option for my daughter?

In the past, underbite was treated by surgically realigning the jaws after the child stopped growing. Now the goal is to avoid surgery whenever possible by intervening when the child is still growing, as young as age 5. If the underbite is confined to the teeth, with no skeletal involvement, braces alone might be enough to correct it. When the underbite is skeletal, caused by the lower jaw outgrowing the upper jaw, surgery can be avoided in children younger than 8. The treatment usually begins with an upper jaw expander, which is a molded plastic and wire device that is fixed to the roof of the mouth and remains in for about a year. Each night for the first few months, the parent uses a key to open the expander slightly. Once the proper jaw width is achieved, the expander remains in place for several more months. After this, it is replaced with a retainer to ensure that the upper jaw hardens in its new position.

At around age 8 or 9, the child may be fitted with a reverse-pull face mask. Resembling a baseball catcher's mask, it is worn after school and at night. The mask is anchored to the mouth with rubber bands, which are attached to metal bands around the top back molars. The gentle but steady pressure exerted by the rubber bands on the upper jaw encourages bone growth and slowly pulls out the upper jaw.

If the underbite is mild or moderate, the lower jaw is left alone. In severe cases, when the growth of the lower jaw needs to be restrained, the child will also wear a chin cap, which wraps around the chin and the top of the head. She wears this cap for as long as necessary for best results; a year is fairly typical. Although the reverse-pull face mask treatment can eliminate the need for surgery, sometimes the discrepancy between the lower and upper jaws is so great that surgery is still needed. After treatment with the face mask or surgery, the child may still need to wear standard braces for one to three years, followed by a retainer for another two years or longer, to achieve and maintain an ideal bite.

The success rates of surgical and nonsurgical correction of an underbite are extremely high. If treatment is started early, most children today can avoid surgery.

CHAPTER 16

Orthodontics

Deciding whether to get braces for your child is a big decision. Just how crooked is crooked, anyway? Do teeth need to be perfectly straight? If your child isn't going to be a movie star, do perfectly aligned teeth matter?

Take a good look at your child, her smile, her teeth alignment, how she looks with mouth open and closed. Does she hide her smile behind her hands? Braces are a decision that will affect your child for the rest of her life. How can you know whether they are a good investment? They are expensive; they can be painful at times; and you won't know the exact results for several years. (Not to mention that once the braces are removed, your child may need to wear a retainer for years to maintain the newly shaped smile.)

The bottom line for her dental and overall health is this: If there's something off about the alignment of your child's teeth or jaws, then it's time to see an orthodontist.

> ### Do Braces Run in the Family?
>
> Some orthodontic problems are genetic. Others develop over time from thumb or finger sucking, mouth breathing, dental disease, accidents, or poor nutrition or dental care. If your child does need braces, take heart! Orthodontics has come a long way since you were young, and your child will probably have a much more pleasant experience than the one you remember.

Orthodontists

Orthodontists are dentists who specialize in straightening teeth and aligning jaws to create optimal function and form. After receiving two additional years of training and education beyond dental school, an orthodontist has learned the skills needed to treat the misalignment of teeth and problems in facial development with braces, headgear, retainers, and other related methods.

Early History of Orthodontics

If you think the desire for straight teeth is something new, think again. Braces date back thousands of years. Archaeologists have discovered mummies from Egypt with crude metal bands around their teeth. In 1728, French dentist Pierre Fauchard published a dental book with an entire chapter devoted to straightening teeth. This was the first evidence of dental research into the topic of orthodontics.

In the early 1900s in America, Edward Angle devised the first simple classification system for malocclusions (bad bites). This system is still used today in modern orthodontics. Dr. Angle simplified many of the appliances used and started the first college for orthodontics in 1901. He also organized the American Society of Orthodontics, which later became the American Academy of Orthodontics, the first specialty in dentistry. These early orthodontists used gold, platinum, and silver to make custom orthodontic appliances. Now we have a clue about why braces cost so much!

The next major advancement in the field occurred in the early 1950s, when orthodontists started using stainless steel to make most orthodontic appliances and the manufacture of orthodontic brackets became standardized. Braces, as they were now called, had bands that wrapped totally around each tooth, and orthodontic appointments were very long by today's standards. Using stainless steel in orthodontics was a significant improvement, in part because the cost was reduced but also because the material was more flexible and easier for the orthodontist to manipulate.

Now fast forward to the 1970s, when direct bonding became a reality in orthodontics. Once braces could be glued, or bonded, directly to the teeth, they got smaller and more presentable. Moreover, these new bonded braces of the 1970s were the beginning of the straight wire techniques still in use today. Straight wire treatment meant orthodontists could spend less time bending wire and thus decrease the time each patient spent in the orthodontic chair. Decreasing how long patients sit in the orthodontic chair is a continuing trend. This is definitely a good thing.

Orthodontics in the Modern Era

Orthodontics has made vast improvements in the past few years, including Invisalign clear plastic aligners, 3-D computer tomography for orthodontic diagnosis, innovative bracket design, orthodontic wires made from a heat-sensitive memory titanium material, and futuristic computer-driven robotic wire bending. Along with these changes came a major rethinking of when and how to treat orthodontic patients.

In the past, orthodontic treatment was usually not started in children until they had lost all their baby teeth and were teenagers, or nearly so. And for many years, teeth were extracted to create space for straightening teeth. Although extractions are still necessary in some situations in orthodontics, they are no longer routine. This change alone has made a whole lot of kids and their parents happy.

Today children are being treated at a much younger age, which can be good for several reasons. Modern orthodontic treatment focuses not only on straightening teeth but also on redirecting the growth of the jaws to help with a child's developing facial structures. This approach to orthodontic care takes into account the growing child's entire face and has improved the treatment of children with problems such as overbites, underbites, and narrow jaw shape. This new approach to orthodontic treatment is called dentofacial orthopedics. Now the American Academy of Orthodontics recommends that children as young as age 7 get an orthodontic evaluation to determine whether they are candidates for this type of early intervention.

A comprehensive orthodontic workup and evaluation is done before the first braces or appliances are placed in your child's mouth. (These workups, which give the orthodontist a road map to correct your child's malocclusion, or bite problems, are described later in this chapter.)

Many companies that make orthodontic braces and appliances spend a lot of money on advertising and marketing both to the public and to orthodontists. But specific brands of orthodontic appliances and braces matter less in the big picture than the orthodontic specialist's experience and treatment techniques. Many orthodontists can show you the results of cases they have treated that are similar to your child's, so you can get an idea of what to expect. Orthodontics is both an art and a science; you'll need to trust the experience of your orthodontic specialist or else get a second opinion.

What is early, or interceptive, orthodontic treatment?

Orthodontic treatment may be recommended and started when your child still has baby teeth, between the ages of 7 and 10. This early orthodontic treatment, also called interceptive, or phase I, treatment, is a fairly recent concept based on addressing certain orthodontic problems before they become worse.

Early treatment is limited to children with significant orthodontic problems, such as underbites, severe crowding, crossbites with narrow jaw shapes, and overbites with protruding teeth that are prone to injury. Many children benefit from this approach, which improves facial appearance, self-esteem, and jaw function. Plus, this early treatment may prevent some dental extractions.

Interceptive treatment is recommended when the same results cannot be achieved if treatment is delayed until all the permanent teeth are in place. Most children can wait until around age 12 before their braces are placed. Everyone wants orthodontic treatment to be both time efficient and cost effective. If your child is between ages 7 and 10, now is the time to ask about how interceptive treatment works and whether your child is a candidate. Phase I treatment usually takes 12 to 18 months. Typically, a second phase of treatment is needed later, after all the permanent teeth come in. This is called phase II.

Why do some children wait until they are older to get braces?

Most orthodontic patients receive only one phase of treatment, called comprehensive treatment, usually beginning around the age of 12. If your child's orthodontic problems do not require early intervention, comprehensive treatment can be delayed until this time. For children who received phase I treatment, phase II is considered part of their comprehensive treatment and begins after a resting period of one to two years between the two phases. This second phase is to make sure that each tooth has an exact location in the mouth and that the bite is correct.

Although the most obvious benefit of comprehensive orthodontic treatment is a beautiful and confident smile, here's a side benefit: straight teeth are easier to clean, which makes them less prone to decay and gum disease later on.

How does the orthodontist know that my child needs braces?

Most orthodontic specialists start with orthodontic records to create a road map for the best possible treatment for each child's situation. Each person's teeth and jaw grow and develop differently. After a child becomes a candidate for orthodontic treatment, the orthodontist considers many factors when putting together a treatment plan. Orthodontic records usually consist of the following.

DENTAL IMPRESSIONS AND MODELS OF THE TEETH

Dental impressions, also known as alginate impressions, are used to obtain an accurate replica of a patient's mouth and teeth by having the child bite into a claylike material. Study models of the mouth are then made by pouring stone into the impression material and allowing it to set. The orthodontist uses the model to study the current position of the child's teeth and to predict the future relationship between the upper and lower teeth. Study models are a permanent record the specialist then has for future reference. More and more orthodontists these days are using a computer 3-D virtual simulation instead of a hard stone model.

PANORAMIC RADIOGRAPH

A panoramic x-ray, also known as a panorex or pan x-ray, is a two-dimensional image of the upper and lower jaws and teeth. This type of x-ray is useful for adolescent patients in particular, because the orthodontist is able to see the developing teeth and predict where they will erupt in the mouth. Children who are experiencing a delay in the eruption of teeth will require this x-ray at an earlier age, to rule out missing or impacted teeth. Adult patients who are considering orthodontic treatment will typically have this x-ray taken for the dentist to see the current health and level of the jawbone and the roots of the teeth.

CEPHALOMETRIC RADIOGRAPH AND CEPHALOMETRIC TRACING

The cephalometric x-ray, or ceph, is an x-ray that captures the side profile of the patient, from the top of the head to just below the tip of the chin. The resulting image includes not only the teeth and bone but also the soft tissues of the face. The orthodontic specialist will use tracing paper or computer imaging to trace the ceph, including important landmarks on the x-ray, to make predictions on how the face and teeth will move during orthodontic treatment. Your child's orthodontist should review this important radiograph with you before treatment is started. New technology called a 3-D cone beam CT scan now allows dental specialists to view facial bones, teeth, and jaw structures in virtual 3-D detail from any angle.

INTRA-ORAL AND FACIAL PHOTOS WITH CLINICAL EXAMINATION

Intra-oral (inside the mouth) and facial photos are taken of the patient's teeth and face. These photos are used to determine the current classification of the child's profile, as well as to provide a permanent record of the orthodontic starting point, to help gauge progress. These images are captured using a digital camera. A clinical examination follows, to assess the child's teeth, gums, TMJ disorder, or any other dental problems before treatment is started.

TREATMENT CONSULTATION

After obtaining all the completed records, the orthodontic specialist notes all potential treatment options in the child's file. At this point, most orthodontists have a consultation with the parents and child to discuss the options. At this consultation, the final treatment plan and fees are agreed on and the appropriate appointments are made.

Getting Braces

The first step in getting braces does not actually involve braces at all. Your child will need to have spacers (or separators) put in. Spacers are small rubber bands stretched and placed around the back teeth to create a little more space between them so that the orthodontist will be able to place orthodontic bands around the molars. Spacers usually stay in place for five to ten days before the braces are placed. At first they feel like pieces of food stuck in between the teeth and may cause some discomfort. Teeth may be sensitive for a few days after receiving spacers, but the spacers must stay in place the entire time.

Here are some guidelines your child should keep in mind while wearing spacers:

> *A Downside of Braces*
>
> Braces provide many benefits, but they also put children at increased risk for cavities. Even the most motivated and diligent child will have difficulty brushing his teeth properly in and among the braces. If you haven't already established a pattern of good oral hygiene, this could be an even bigger problem. Talk to the dentist or orthodontist about how your child's current dental habits might affect the safety of getting braces. To get the most out of the braces and ensure your child's long-term oral health, always be honest and work with your child's dental care providers toward the best solution for your family.

- Do not pick at the spacers with your fingers or tongue.
- Do not floss the teeth where the spacers are placed.
- Avoid sticky foods that may pull out the spacers.
- Take a pain reliever if needed.
- Let your orthodontist know if any of the spacers have fallen out so that they can be replaced.

The day the braces are placed is a big day. The process may take an hour or so, depending on whether your child is getting both top and bottom braces placed on the same day or just the top braces. The spacers are removed, and bands will be fit to the correct size for your child's molars. The bands are then cemented to the back teeth with tooth cement.

The rest of the braces will be bonded to each tooth with a special glue that only hardens after being exposed to a bright blue light. First, a plastic lip separator is usually placed to keep lips and tongue away from the braces as they are being placed, because any moisture during placement will prevent the brackets from setting securely. Then the teeth are thoroughly cleaned with a gritty pumice material, rinsed, and dried.

A mild acid etching agent is placed on the teeth next, before a sealer is painted over the bracket, which has been specifically designed with the correct angles and tips to help guide the tooth to the correct position. How the bracket is positioned on the tooth is an important step. Your child's orthodontist will take time to place the braces on the teeth with a high degree of precision.

After the braces have been placed, the next step is attaching the arch wire, which is what moves the teeth over time. Each bracket has a horizontal slot

---

The Language of Braces

Here are some common words used to describe the parts of the braces:

Arch wire: The main wire for moving teeth. It comes in different sizes and thicknesses.

Bands: The metal rings that fit around the tooth to anchor an appliance or braces in the back of the mouth.

Brackets: Small metal parts that hold the wire for the braces. Brackets are bonded to the teeth and are what the beige or colored elastics are placed on.

Elastics: Tiny beige or colored elastic O-rings that hold the arch wire to the brackets.

Hooks: What the rubber bands are attached to.

Ligatures: Small metal wires that hold the arch wire to the brackets.

Power chain: Elastic chains that close spaces.

Rubber bands: Bands that help move the teeth in the desired direction.

Spacers (separators): Small rubber bands that are flossed between the back teeth to create space to fit the orthodontic bands around the molars.

Ties: Same as elastics.

for the wire, which then is either held in place by a colored elastic O-ring or snapped into place by a locking spring on the brackets (this is called self-ligation). Once the arch wire is positioned, your child will be given instructions on how to care for these expensive little teeth jewels.

No part of this process is particularly painful, but sitting for a long time can be boring for your child and having to keep her mouth open is uncomfortable. Once the arch wire begins to move the teeth, your child will feel some pressure and discomfort, which can usually be relieved with a mild pain medicine like Tylenol or Advil. The teeth are moved into the desired location by applying a mild continuous pressure to the teeth over time. The farther they have to move, the longer the treatment will take.

Are there different kinds of braces?

Most people think of braces as metal brackets bonded to teeth and connected by a wire held in place with colored rubber O-rings. But there is another approach. In 1997 Zia Chishti co-founded Align Technology, a 3-D computer-imaging technology company that produced a proprietary method of orthodontic treatment using a series of clear removable aligners as an alternative to the traditional metal brace. The technique is called Invisalign Orthodontics.

With Invisalign Orthodontics and their similar competitors, patients wear computer-designed vacuum-formed plastic aligners full time, as they would a retainer. A new aligner is delivered by the dentist every two to three weeks and is worn to achieve an incremental change in your teeth. These aligners only work when worn consistently, so the patient needs to be fully committed to the treatment. The aligners are removed only during eating and tooth brushing. There are no eating restrictions while wearing Invisalign.

As a relatively new technique, Invisalign treatment has gone through many improvements and refinements, and more and more people are being treated with this technique, including some older teenagers. Most children, especially those with complex orthodontic problems, are not candidates for Invisalign treatment. If your orthodontic specialist advises you against the treatment for your child, he or she almost certainly has good reasons for doing so.

What are self-ligating braces and how are they different from traditional braces?

With traditional braces, the arch wire is held in place by small rubber O-rings called ties or small metal wires called ligatures. Self-ligating braces hold the wire in place with a locking clip or sliding door. Self-ligating braces are reported to have some advantages over traditional braces, including low friction between the brackets and arch wire, resulting in quicker tooth movement with less force on the teeth. The arch wire can be removed and replaced more quickly, which means shorter orthodontic appointments. Remember, this is a theme of modern orthodontic practice: short appointments. Self-ligation is also considered more hygienic and less uncomfortable than traditional brackets.

These advantages have not yet been fully confirmed scientifically, although results are promising. Orthodontic manufacturers promote their products over the competition with major advertising campaigns. Some of the self-ligating products you will see advertised are SmartClip, by 3M, In-Ovation, by Densply, and Damon, by Ormco. Trust your child's orthodontic specialist's technique and product choices, or get a second opinion.

What are ceramic, or tooth-colored, braces?

Ceramic brackets are made of a tooth-colored translucent ceramic material. They are strong and generally do not stain. Most orthodontists charge a premium to use ceramic brackets. Many people choose ceramic because they blend in with the teeth and are less noticeable than metal brackets. These are the type of braces many celebrities have as adults. Ceramic braces are actually harder than tooth enamel and therefore could possibly wear away enamel if you were to grind your teeth against the brackets. For that reason they are sometimes not used on the lower teeth.

The newer versions of ceramic braces use the self-ligation technique, so they do not require rubber O-ring ties, which can stain.

What are lingual braces?

Lingual braces are placed behind the teeth and are therefore all but invisible to everyone. Lingual braces require extra training to place, so not every orthodontist offers them, and they are mostly reserved for adults. Most orthodontists charge more for lingual braces because they take more time to adjust. Because they are placed on the tongue side of the mouth, lingual braces affect speech more than traditional braces do and tend to irritate the tongue, so they are not advisable for everyone.

Other Orthodontic Treatments

Do orthodontists use anything other than braces?

Along with traditional braces, orthodontists use many other appliances to move the teeth and jaws during treatment. You'd almost think that an orthodontist would need a degree in mechanical engineering to figure out how to use all these appliances. For years orthodontists have struggled with choosing between appliances that require patient cooperation and that can be removed and possibly lost and appliances that are fixed to the teeth and do not require much cooperation.

Headgear, palatal expanders, quad helix, Herbst, Forsus, Bionator, and Twin Block are just a few of the orthodontic and orthopedic appliances orthodontists use to widen or realign the jaws for a better bite. These appliances are used in growing children to achieve the desired results, which is why timing in orthodontics can be important. Some are used to align the jaws by moving the lower jaw and teeth forward or the upper jaw and teeth backward. Some are removable, but most are fixed to the teeth. Orthodontists tend to rely on two or three appliances that work best in their hands. These preferences come from years of experience using appliances.

Palatal expanders have been used for years with good results to correct crossbites and narrow upper arches. RPE is one type of palatal expander that has an expansion screw placed in the palate to widen the arch. The parent adjusts the child's expander each day until the correct arch width is achieved, after which the expander must stay in place for months, to allow bone to form and to stabilize the correction.

Headgear is a removable appliance worn to restrict growth of the upper jaw and improve an overbite problem. It consists of a wire facebow that attaches to the upper molars and a strap that fits around the neck or head. Headgear works well, but only if the child is cooperative and wears it correctly.

A Herbst appliance is fixed to the teeth and is worn to help correct an overbite condition of the jaws. It is designed to advance the lower jaw and works only in a growing child. One of the newest appliances is the Forsus, which is similar to the Herbst. The Forsus advances the lower jaw and teeth into a better relationship and is fixed to the teeth, so it does not require the patient's cooperation.

What are temporary anchorage devices and how are they used in orthodontics?

Temporary anchorage devices, known as TADs or mini-screws, have dramatically altered what orthodontists can do without jaw surgery. TADs are tiny titanium screws placed in the palate or gum area to serve as a stabilizing point to move teeth. The mini-screw is removed after the desired tooth movement is achieved. In orthodontics, teeth are moved by pitting larger or more teeth (the anchor or anchorage) against smaller or fewer teeth. But as Newton taught us, for each force there is an equal and opposite force that sometimes works against orthodontists in moving teeth effectively. TADs address this problem by providing a stable anchor, enabling orthodontists to treat extraordinarily difficult malocclusions in a simpler way. Most of the time these mini-screws are placed with only a topical anesthetic rubbed on the gums to provide some numbing.

What is orthognathic jaw surgery?

Orthognathic surgery, or jaw surgery, is considered by the orthodontist only when the bite problem is so severe that orthodontic treatment alone will not correct the problem. The purposes of jaw surgery are to correct an underlying skeletal problem caused by the dysfunctional bite and to address concerns about appearance. Orthognathic jaw surgery may also be considered as part of treatment for obstructive sleep apnea. Orthognathic jaw surgery is rarely advised in growing children, because the hope is that conventional orthodontic and dentofacial orthopedic treatment can correct the underlying problem. If orthognathic surgery is considered as part of a comprehensive treatment plan for your child, then an oral maxillofacial surgeon will be consulted before any treatment is started.

Orthodontic Treatment Costs

At first glance, braces seem expensive, but consider that this treatment may take several years and a lot of valuable time from an experienced orthodontist and staff. The average cost of orthodontic treatment is between $3,000 and $6,000, depending on where you live and what needs to be done. Treatment is usually more costly in major cities than in rural areas. There may be an additional charge for the orthodontic records, or workup, before the braces are placed.

Because treatment lasts one to three years (with two years being the average), most orthodontic specialists offer a payment plan option. When treatment is started, a down payment is usually collected, equaling 20 to 30 percent of the total treatment fees. The balance is paid over the course of treatment. You will usually be presented with a detailed contract to sign that spells out your financial responsibility. This document should also describe any extra fees, including charges for missed appointments or broken appliances and retainers if these are not included in the total treatment cost. Read the contract before treatment is started. These fees can add up. Some offices offer a discount for paying the total amount of treatment up front.

Will my insurance cover my child's orthodontics?

Orthodontic insurance may cover part of the cost of orthodontics. Understand your coverage before seeking treatment. Orthodontic insurance coverage works differently than dental insurance does. Most orthodontic plans have a lifetime maximum benefit the insurer will pay. The payout is usually a percentage of the treatment fees, usually around 50 percent over the course of treatment until the maximum is met. If you pay for the total treatment up front, don't expect your insurance to reimburse you the total amount up front. Some insurance companies pay one amount if you have treatment performed by an in-network orthodontic specialist they have contracted with and a lesser amount to anyone else out of network. Some orthodontic offices will arrange to accept payments directly from your insurance company and will ask you to pay your portion, and other offices will ask you to pay for your treatment and have the insurance company reimburse you. Most insurance companies pay orthodontic benefits every three months instead of monthly.

In a perfect world, your child will start and finish treatment with the same orthodontic specialist. If you move before treatment is completed, however, and a new orthodontist has to finish, your total fees will almost certainly increase. The new orthodontist needs to assess the treatment progress, create new records, and work up a new treatment plan. There may be a course change as well. The new orthodontist will usually charge for retainers separately.

Living with Braces

Whether your child has just gotten braces or has just had them tightened, they can be tough on his teeth. The key is to help him be gentle with his mouth. If you just had a good long workout, how would you feel? Tired, sore, and achy. Well, that's how teeth feel right after orthodontic work! Here are some tips for your child to minimize the pain of tender teeth:

- Stay away from chewy and sticky foods and eat foods that are soft, such as yogurt, ripened and sliced fruit, smoothies and milkshakes, pudding, gelatin, macaroni and cheese, and soup.
    - Eat slowly and carefully.
    - If it hurts to chew something, don't! It will only make your mouth hurt worse. Better yet, don't chew at all. Try mashing the food by pressing it against the roof of your mouth with your tongue. If you need to chew, use your back teeth.

> *Recipes for Braces*
>
> Collect some recipes that you can make on tooth-tender days so you're prepared to offer maximum nutritional value with as little chewing as possible. Pamela Waterman and Amee Hoge's Braces Cookbook 2 (www.metalmouthmedia.net) includes many great recipes.

How should my child take care of her braces?

To have a successful outcome with braces, your child should be an active partner in caring for them. Her cooperation plays a major part in her orthodontic treatment. Thankfully, taking care of braces is not complicated. It can be broken down into two basic categories: good dental hygiene and following the proper diet.

Dental plaque is the number one enemy to anyone wearing braces. It can cause tooth decay, gum disease, and bad breath. No one wants to have straight teeth with ugly spots on them after their braces are removed. An electric toothbrush may make cleaning her teeth easier, but it is not necessary. A soft-bristled manual toothbrush works just fine. A travel toothbrush may be helpful to take to school and keep in her backpack or locker. She will need to clean her teeth after each meal and before bedtime, paying special attention to the area between the braces and gum tissue. It helps to focus on a few teeth at a time and make sure they are perfectly clean before moving on to the next area. Your child should be sure to brush along the gum line as well as on the teeth. If a fluoride rinse is recommended to prevent

> *Take Good Care!*
>
> Any orthodontic appliance, including braces and retainers, is carefully engineered and made up of many tiny parts. Although they are tough, they aren't indestructible. In fact, there has never been any type of orthodontic appliance that some kids are not able to destroy. So ask your child to please be careful.

dental decay, your child should follow her orthodontist's advice about using it.

A proxabrush is a small pointed brush used to clean between the orthodontic wire and gum tissue. Using the proxabrush gently is important to avoid damaging the braces or hurting her gums. A Waterpik can help loosen food and plaque before brushing or flossing, but it does not take the place of good tooth brushing. Dental floss is your child's friend while wearing braces. Flossing with braces may take a little longer, but it is well worth it in the long run. It can help keep the gums from becoming inflamed and swollen during treatment. Using a threader can help get the floss around the braces.

In addition to keeping her teeth and gums clean and healthy at home, going to the dentist for regular cleanings is important. Her dentist can check for dental decay or gum problems before they become serious. If the teeth are not kept clean during orthodontic treatment, plaque left around the braces can decalcify the enamel, creating discolored areas called white spot lesions. These discolorations may become permanent white halos around the areas where the brackets were bonded on the teeth.

What foods should my son avoid with braces?

Some offices charge an extra fee for broken or dislodged brackets that need to be rebonded. Common sense will tell your child how to avoid damaging his braces. Hard foods like nuts, candied apples, and taffy peanut brittle can break or damage wires and brackets. Foods like corn on the cob can be a problem. Bagels can be chewy and hard on braces (and difficult to chew after an adjustment to braces).

Sticky foods like chewing gum, gummy bears, and Fruit Roll-Ups get caught between the brackets. Sugary foods and candies cause tooth decay and enamel decalcification (white spots on teeth). Biting his fingernails or chewing on objects like pencils can break his braces. Perhaps above all, your child should avoid chewing ice.

Can my child play sports with braces on?

Your child can still play sports while wearing braces, but she'll need to wear a mouth guard to protect her teeth and the braces. Let her orthodontist know if you need help deciding on the best mouth guard for the type of appliance she is wearing. There are two basic styles of sports mouth guards: the ones that are already formed and shaped and the ones that are boiled and molded to the teeth. Both styles will work, but comfort is an important part of the formula. (For more information about mouth guards, see chapter 18, "Dental Trauma and Emergencies.")

What should we do if there's a problem with the braces?

Braces are extremely useful in helping to create gorgeous new smiles, but they can be difficult to maintain. Braces, bands, and wires sometimes break or fall off. Usually this is caused by chewing hard or sticky foods or by some type of trauma to the mouth. More often, one of the parts will just come loose. Here are a few common problems and suggested solutions.

LOOSE OR BROKEN BRACKET (BRACE)

The braces (also called brackets) are the metal or ceramic pieces that are attached to the teeth. They're usually attached using a material called composite resin. It is similar to the tooth-colored material used for some fillings. Chewing something hard or sticky can weaken or break the resin. When that happens, a brace can come loose. It may poke into your child's gums, tongue, or cheek. Regardless of how the brace broke, call the orthodontist right away to have it repaired.

When your child's braces were first put on, his orthodontist will have given him some dental, or orthodontic, wax. Your child can put the wax over the bracket to keep it from poking until he can see his orthodontist.

LOOSE BAND

Bands are the metal rings that are cemented around back teeth (and sometimes around front teeth). If a band becomes loose, call for an appointment to have it recemented or replaced. If the band comes off completely, do not try to put it back on. Save it and bring it to your child's appointment.

PROTRUDING OR BROKEN WIRE

If a wire breaks or sticks out, it can hurt the cheek, tongue, or gum. Your child may be able to use the eraser end of a pencil to push the wire into a better position. If that doesn't work, she can put a small piece of orthodontic wax over the end of the wire. Do not cut the wire. A cut wire can be accidentally swallowed or inhaled. If the wire has caused a sore, have your child rinse her mouth with warm saltwater or an antiseptic rinse. Rinsing will keep the area clean and reduce discomfort. She can also use an over-the-counter topical oral pain reliever to temporarily numb the area until she can see her orthodontist.

RUBBER BAND PROBLEMS

A rubber band left in the mouth too long can snap and be painful. If rubber bands are left off completely for too long, the braces may need to stay on longer. Changing rubber bands on braces is not hard. Talk to your child's orthodontist about how often they need to be changed.

If your child accidentally swallows a rubber band, don't worry. The rubber band is safe to swallow unless he is allergic to it. The band just passes through his digestive system and comes out in a bowel movement.

Broken or loose brackets, bands, or wires take time to repair. The orthodontist may adjust, reposition, or reattach the existing wires or brackets or completely replace brackets or wires. If your child does not have any discomfort and the problem does not interfere with treatment, the orthodontist may delay major repairs until the next regular appointment. In any case, call the office before that appointment to make sure enough time is scheduled to complete the repairs.

How are the braces removed?

Braces are removed with a special instrument that breaks the bond between the bracket and the enamel of the tooth. The orthodontist will then clean away the remaining bonding with a dental polisher. This will make the surface of the teeth feel very smooth compared to the feeling of braces on the teeth. Fluoride is usually applied at this time. New impressions of your child's teeth will be taken so the orthodontist can make custom retainers for her to wear.

What are retainers and why are they important?

Orthodontic retainers are custom-made devices, usually of plastic and wires, to hold teeth in position after braces. Most people need to wear some type of retainer after braces.

There are three different retainers orthodontists prescribe. The classic is the Hawley retainer, with colored plastic material on the inside of the teeth and a wire on the front. The Hawley has been used for many years. The advantage of this type of retainer is that the metal wire can be adjusted to make minor adjustments to the front teeth if needed.

Another popular retainer used by orthodontists is the invisible vacuum-formed Essix retainer. This transparent retainer fits over the entire dental arch, much like Invisalign trays. Essix retainers are less expensive to make and less conspicuous, and most people say they are easier to wear than Hawley retainers. The Essix may be right for a person who grinds his teeth because it will protect the enamel from wear. After a while, however, if the bruxism (or grinding), wears away the plastic retainer, it will need to be replaced.

During the first few days of wearing a retainer, your child may experience extra saliva in his mouth, and his speech may be affected. Both of these problems will go away after a few days, as he gets used to wearing the retainer.

An entirely different category of retainers are fixed, or bonded, retainers. A fixed retainer is a small wire bonded to the tongue side of the teeth. This type of retainer is more commonly used on the lower teeth than the upper and is more likely to be prescribed if the lower teeth were crooked before treatment. The advantage of this retainer is that it is permanently fixed to the teeth. The drawback is that it is difficult to floss around, and tartar may build up around it. Just like with braces, floss threaders help to pass dental floss under the wire and between the teeth.

Retainers that aren't fixed are worn for 10 to 20 hours a day as prescribed by the orthodontist. Your child will need one for many years after the braces are removed, to keep the teeth in position. Our teeth continue to move ever so slightly as we age. (Plastic surgeons wish they had retainers to help preserve their treatment results!)

The Future of Orthodontics

The future of orthodontics looks bright. As technology enhances our daily lives, it also continues to advance the science of orthodontics. More and more companies are using computers and digital imaging to make orthodontic treatment more precise and faster. For example, the Sure-Smile System by OraMetrix takes 3-D images of a patient's teeth and helps the orthodontist develop a precise treatment plan to move teeth more effectively, which will reduce the time in braces. The company makes individualized custom arch wires for the patient using robotic machines. As other companies develop more precise high-tech material and methods, braces will be worn for a shorter time, will be smaller and less visible, and will produce less discomfort and give better results.

These developments have changed how orthodontics is done—and that's something to smile about. Orthodontia will always be part science and part art, with both parts equally important.

CHAPTER 17

Tooth Appearance

Stains, spots, and missing teeth can detract from even the most adorable grin. Teeth problems have a way of drawing attention to themselves. What can be done? Your child's dentist can help fix and prevent problems. Your role is to prevent and notice potential problems and get your child to a dentist quickly.

Tooth Stains

Many parents wonder why their young children's teeth are stained. Some causes are internal, and some causes are external. Stains that come from within the tooth itself have a few potential causes:

- *Medications.* The antibiotic tetracycline, if taken during pregnancy, can cause a child to have discolored baby teeth as can other medications and supplements, especially those containing iron.
- *Excessive fluoride.* Too much fluoride may cause bright white spots or streaks on the teeth.
- *Newborn jaundice.* A baby who develops jaundice after birth may have teeth come in with a green tint.
- *Serious illness.* Infections during infancy, hepatitis, and some types of heart disease may discolor the baby teeth.

What Is Hypocalcification?

A tooth disturbed while it is being formed may develop atypical enamel, which usually appears as a white, yellow, or brown discoloration on one or more surfaces of the tooth. This most commonly affects the first permanent molars and the two front teeth, although it can happen to any tooth. In mild forms, it shows as white marks on the teeth, usually near the chewing edge, but it may be anywhere on your child's tooth. The marks are often hydration dependent, meaning that if the tooth dries out, white spots become more prominent. When the tooth remains wet, the spots diminish or disappear.

White blemishes that are large and opaque will likely need to be removed and the blemished area filled with a cosmetic filling material. Yellow or brown spots are often improved with bleaching.

Teeth can become discolored from extrinsic factors, on the outside, as well:

• *Inadequate brushing.* If teeth aren't brushed properly, plaque may form on the teeth, which can lead to yellow tooth discoloration.

• *Tooth or gum injury.* Trauma to teeth or gums may cause discoloration, often a pink or gray tint.

Why does my son have a black spot on his tooth?

Black spots can occur anywhere on teeth—front teeth or molars. Reasons for a black spot include a stained pit or fissure in the tooth. Food debris or stains can accumulate within the fissure or the pit and turn the area black. People who eat a lot of sweets can develop black spots in fissures if they do not clean their teeth regularly. Some of these spots are harmless—just crud that builds up in the fissure—but other spots are a sign that a small cavity is developing. Some old silver fillings can take on a blackish discoloration, which isn't a big concern. Ramp up the oral hygiene and ask the dentist to check it out at your child's next checkup.

Black or brown stains are sometimes caused by trauma. If a child's tooth is hit, the blood vessels inside the tooth hemorrhage and cause the blood to enter the dentin layer (just beneath the enamel). This results in a discolored tooth. After trauma to the tooth, discoloration may not show immediately. Your child needs to see the dentist soon after tooth trauma.

My child's teeth have white or yellow spots on them. What causes this?

When new teeth erupt, they may have small (or large) white spots on them. These spots, formed during development, are called enamel hypoplasia, or hypocalcification. The color defects in the teeth can range from milky white to yellow or brown. Sometimes the enamel, or outer layer of the tooth, is underdeveloped or thin in places. These white or yellow spots are common. In baby teeth, they can appear on the very back molars. In adult teeth, the first permanent molars are often affected. Whitish or brownish chalky spots are usually caused by too much fluoride during a child's early years. Spotted front teeth often raise concerns about appearance.

What is swimmer's tooth?

Children who swim competitively, particularly those who swim more than 6 hours per week, may be at risk for developing yellowish brown or dark brown stains on their teeth, often called swimmer's tooth. Because of the time they spend in the pool, these children expose their teeth to large amounts of chemically treated water, which has a higher pH than saliva. This change in pH causes proteins in the saliva to break down and form hard, brown tartarlike deposits on the teeth, usually the front teeth. To prevent this, many dentists recommend that athlete swimmers come in for regular cleanings and dental visits more often than twice a year.

Can High Fevers Cause Tooth Damage?

If a child has a high fever for a long period before the age of 10, damage to the permanent teeth can occur. When the adult teeth come in, there may be markings across the teeth that were developing during the time of the fever. Markings may appear anywhere on the teeth, from faint lines or ridges all the way to a badly damaged tooth. Also, the strength of the enamel may have been compromised, making the teeth more susceptible to decay. Your child's dentist will probably notice the damage during an exam and may ask you about any history of high fevers. Treatment depends on how severe the problem is and where it is located—and how much it bothers your child.

Should children have their teeth whitened?

Children want nice-looking teeth and can be self-conscious about dental stains and discolorations. Although tooth bleaching and aesthetic dentistry are available for children over age 12, these products and procedures can be problematic. About 60 percent of children using tooth-whitening products suffer from gum irritation and teeth sensitivity. In fact, whitening that uses bleaching combined with light can cause pulp damage in children under 18. Also, children who continue the practice throughout their lives could overwhiten, causing the teeth to eventually become gray.

You may want to consider making some changes to your child's eating habits to prevent teeth from becoming yellowed or stained rather than focusing on quick tooth-whitening treatments that could damage your child's teeth. Whitening toothpaste and gum are other inexpensive and mild solutions.

Should children get veneers?

Porcelain veneers, also called dental veneers, dental porcelain, or porcelain laminates, are a form of cosmetic dentistry aimed at placing a custom-fitted wafer-thin porcelain shell over or around the tooth to mask its imperfections. Held in place by bonding agents, the veneer adheres directly to the tooth's enamel, making the porcelain stronger. The color of veneers can be matched to the other teeth, making them hardly noticeable.

Porcelain veneers are for aesthetic purposes and should be used only on permanent teeth. Veneers cannot be used to cover unhealthy teeth, such as those affected by tooth decay and gum disease. They also tend to chip and break easily, so they aren't ideal for young or active children or kids who grind their teeth.

Ancient Tooth Whitening

The practice of tooth whitening began around 4,000 years ago with the Egyptians, who created a whitening paste using ground pumice stone mixed with wine vinegar. White teeth were a mark of beauty and a sign of wealth. Ancient Romans whitened their teeth using urine. Yes, urine. The ammonia in the urine was the bleaching agent. In the seventeenth century, people relied on their barbers for the care of hair and teeth. The barber (who served as the local dentist at the time) would file down the teeth and apply an acid that would whiten them. Although the practice made teeth look whiter, it eroded tooth enamel and led to decay.

Before choosing veneers for your child, find out about the dentist's methods. Ideally, you want the dentist to remove as little enamel or dentin as possible before the veneer is adhered to the tooth. This way, if the veneers need to be removed later, there is little tooth damage underneath. Overall, with porcelain veneers, more of the original tooth and enamel are preserved than with other procedures, such as crowns.

Other Treatments to Improve Appearance

The edges of my child's teeth seem jagged. Can I get them sanded down?

Newly erupted front teeth have bumpy biting edges called mamelons. The mamelons are part of normal tooth anatomy and usually wear away with chewing. If they don't go away, your child's dentist can file down and smooth out the jagged sharp edges of the teeth. Dental shaping (or filing) is the least expensive method of fixing sharp or jagged front teeth.

Can my daughter have her gums recontoured?

Some people have too much gum tissue; it covers their teeth and gives them a gummy smile. Other people have uneven gums that are not scalloped up and down properly. Children naturally have an excess amount of gums, which normally recedes at puberty. The receding, called passive eruption, does not happen in 10 percent of people. Although your child's gums may not be picture perfect yet, don't consider gum contouring until the end of adolescence. Talk to your child's dentist about your concerns, and if it needs to be done, gum recontouring can be done by laser. This method is effective, safe, and efficient, but your child may have temporary minor swelling or discomfort. This pain can be eased with over-the-counter pain medications.

What are flippers?

A dental flipper is the least expensive way to temporarily replace a missing tooth usually costing about $100 to $300. Dental flippers are used by many children in beauty pageants and by child actors and models. The flipper is made by taking an impression of the mouth, and then pouring a plaster cast. An acrylic tooth is selected that most closely matches the shade of the teeth, and a pink plate is molded to fit the child's palate (to replace an upper tooth) or to fit just inside the tongue side of the teeth (to replace a lower tooth), similar to a retainer. Depending on how much you want to spend, there are several variations of flippers available that may look or feel more natural.

Although a dental flipper is meant to be temporary, some people wear them for years. Flippers are not very healthy for the gums, however, because they wear on them. They also break easily and can make eating difficult. When they are not strong enough to eat with, they have to be removed for meals.

Crowns

A crown, or a tooth-shaped cap, is a cover placed over the entire tooth. Crowns can be used on any teeth, including molars and front teeth, either primary or permanent teeth.

Adults usually require several visits to have crowns placed, but for children, the process is much simpler, sometimes requiring only a single visit. Dentists will use a crown for a child when

- the tooth has extensive decay, often on multiple sides
- the child with significant decay also has poor oral hygiene habits
- a filling would be large, weakening the tooth and making it more likely to break
- a tooth is considered weak because it did not develop normally or because it has been broken or undergone root canal therapy
- the tooth is misshapen or discolored and this appearance is concerning

What are crowns made of?

With children, several different kinds of crowns can be customized to fit any tooth. Stainless steel crowns are the most common, especially for primary teeth and molars. These crowns have been used in children for fifty years and are durable, which is important since children tend to be rough on their teeth. However, many parents don't like the look of them, particularly on teeth that are visible. Some steel crowns have a white coating on the front to make them look more "tooth-like," but they are harder to place than regular stainless steel crowns and the white coating can chip off.

Strip crowns are made using a clear form that is filled with plastic material and placed over the tooth. After light curing, the outer clear shell is removed, leaving a white filling completely surrounding the tooth. This allows the tooth to look more natural. Strip crowns are fragile, though, and their durability depends on how much tooth is left and how well the tooth was prepared for the crown. They also take longer to place than stainless steel crowns, and injury to the tooth can break, loosen, or dislodge this type of crown. Similar to the strip crown process, dentists can place a white plastic shell around the tooth, but many do not prefer these types of crowns since children tend to chew through the plastic, causing more problems.

The porcelain crowns most adults are used to can only be used on permanent teeth. Baby teeth are too small for them.

How are crowns put in?

The dentist will first rub an anesthetic gel or cream on a small area of the gum or inner cheek. Once the area is numb, the dentist will inject a local anesthetic. This will numb the area of the mouth where the crown will be placed. Then a dental drill is used to remove the decay and to shape the tooth so that the crown will fit over it. Next, the dentist will reduce the chewing surface of the tooth, and then the sides that touch other teeth. The smallest possible crown is placed, although it must touch the neighboring teeth to help keep them in line and prevent problems in the bite.

Once the tooth is prepared, the next steps depend on the type of crown. The dentist will test any fabricated crown to make sure it fits the tooth. Then the crown will be shaped to fit as closely as possible. Your child's dentist may also and shape a mold (called a crown form) for the tooth first. After the crown is shaped to fit the tooth, it will be polished and filled with cement, then pushed into place on the tooth and further shaped. Any extra cement or plastic will be removed, then the dentist will rinse your child's mouth and examine the tooth and surrounding area, especially to make sure the bite is correct.

Pay attention if your child complains that her teeth don't come together right or that biting "feels funny." The crown may need to be checked to make sure it is not uneven with the other teeth. At each dental examination, your child's dentist will check to make sure the crown is still in place, has not become loose, and has not been damaged. Your child may have some mild discomfort after a crown is placed. This is usually caused by irritation of the tooth's pulp or the soft tissue around the tooth. The discomfort typically goes away after the first 24 hours. If your child complains of pain for several days, contact the dentist's office. Over-the-counter pain medicines can help.

Dental Trauma and Emergencies

Split lips, cut tongues, chipped teeth—all par for the course with children. Fortunately, mouth injuries (even the really bloody ones) are usually minor and easily treated. Here's what you need to know to prevent and treat mouth injuries in your child.

What to Do about a Mouth Injury

Most mouth injuries in children look much worse than they are. There are so many blood vessels in the head and neck that even a tiny cut on your little one's lip or tongue can cause a lot of bleeding. Even figuring out where all that blood is coming from can be hard, and it's bound to be a little scary (especially if you're the weak-kneed type), but try to stay calm. Chances are, you're dealing with a minor injury. Plus, the calmer you are, the faster your child will calm down. Then follow these steps to reduce the bleeding, ease the pain, prevent infection, and start the healing of a mouth injury:

1. *Stop the bleeding.* For bleeding from the outer lip or tongue, apply gentle pressure to the area with a piece of gauze or a clean cloth (run it first under cool water if possible) for as long as you are able (10 minutes of pressure is ideal but may not be realistic if you have a squirming baby or toddler on your

hands). For bleeding from the inner lip (upper or lower), gently press the part of the lip that's bleeding against your child's teeth (or gums) for 10 minutes (or, again, as long as you're able, given the wriggling). Avoid pulling the lip away to check out the damage—that will start the bleeding again.

2. *Distract as you treat.* If there were ever a time to put on a favorite DVD or pull out a favorite distraction, this would be it. The longer your child sits (relatively) still for treatment, the sooner the bleeding will stop.

3. *Keep it cool.* To numb the pain and reduce the swelling, apply an ice pack (or a bag of frozen peas) to the cheek area with a towel or cloth between the cold and the skin to avoid irritation. Sucking on a Popsicle is a cool way to soothe a minor mouth injury.

4. *Provide pain relief as needed.* Most mouth injuries don't keep a child down for long, but if your child seems to be in a lot of discomfort, a dose of acetaminophen or ibuprofen (if he's over age 6 months) should ease the pain. The pain and swelling often reach their peak 24 to 48 hours after the trauma and should gradually improve after that.

5. *Feed with care.* While the cut is on the mend, a diet on the bland side is best. Anything salty or acidic, like orange juice, may sting. If the cut is inside the mouth, a softer-than-usual diet may irritate less. Popsicles will continue to be a soothing treat. Rinsing with warm water after meals (if that skill has been mastered) will keep food from accumulating in a mouth cut.

6. *Give it a few days.* Minor mouth injuries in children (and again, most are minor) usually heal in three to four days. Baby teeth are notorious for developing a dental abscess (infection) after trauma, so be on the lookout for increased swelling, pain, and redness.

When should you call the doctor about a mouth injury?

You can treat most mouth injuries in children at home, but be sure to call the doctor under any of these circumstances:

- Heavy bleeding that doesn't stop, especially after 10 minutes of direct pressure
- Deep or gaping cut that may need stitches

- Embedded debris or dirt in the wound, especially if it was caused by a dirty or rusty object
- Any puncture wound (caused by falling on something pointed like a pen, pencil, or nail, for example)
  - Animal or human bites
  - Injury to the bone
  - Broken or knocked-out tooth (call the dentist first)
- Signs of infection (redness, increased swelling and pain, or unexplained fever)

What should we do when an emergency happens after our dentist's office is closed?

First, don't panic. Dental emergencies are common. Unfortunately, as we all know from experience, they tend to happen at the most inappropriate times, such as on Saturday, in the middle of the night, or while we're on vacation. Call your child's dentist right away after the injury has happened. Most dentists have an after-hours call service that will talk you through what to do in case of an emergency. For a non-life-threatening (or non-tooth-threatening) issue, many temporary solutions will work for a day or two until your child can see a dentist. Even if you think an injury is minor, it is still important to connect with your child's dentist as soon as possible to prevent any long-term damage.

If you cannot reach your child's dentist, go to the hospital emergency room. If your child experiences unconsciousness, bleeding that will not stop, intense pain, or broken bones or teeth, *go to the emergency room immediately.* Always check back with your child's dentist soon after the emergency has been treated and stabilized.

Can mouth injuries be prevented?

No matter how many precautions you take, or rules you set and enforce, you won't be able to prevent every mouth injury. Still, they'll happen less often with some basic preventive measures:

- Childproof your home by getting rid of slippery rugs and protecting sharp edges on furniture and fireplaces to discourage slips and soften those inevitable falls.

- Carefully supervise play at pools, playgrounds, and anywhere it is easy for your child to jump or fall and bump her mouth and teeth.

- Don't let your child walk or run while holding a sharp object, toy, pencil, or toothbrush in or near her mouth.

- Make sure your child sits down quietly while eating, even snacking. Serve smaller portions of food, making it easier to chew slowly and carefully.

- Be vigilant about your child wearing a helmet when riding a bike, scooter, or horse.

- Always properly secure your baby or toddler in a car seat.

> ### Toothpicks
>
> Toothpicks have a long history, dating back to 3500 BC, but they are less than ideal for cleaning teeth. Over 8,000 injuries a year happen with toothpicks, most of them in the mouths of children under age 14. Toothpicks can easily hurt tender gum, tongue, and cheek tissue, and pieces of toothpick can be swallowed, leading to infection and emergency surgery. Plus, researchers have found a rare gum disease caused by toothpicks made from trees infected with Dutch Elm disease. Play it safe and keep toothpicks out of reach of children.

My son just fell and hit his mouth. Should I be worried about his teeth?

Active young children naturally get bumps and bruises—including trauma to their primary teeth (baby teeth). Most accidents to baby teeth *look* bad, but many of them don't need to be seen by a doctor. Swelling is to be expected and may look worse 12 to 24 hours after the injury.

Teeth are remarkably strong, but they aren't indestructible. They can chip, crack (fracture), or break when a person

- bites down on something hard
- is hit in the face or mouth
- falls down
- has cavities that weaken the tooth

My daughter fell and bumped her tooth a few weeks ago.
It didn't get loose, but now the tooth is brown! What can I do?

Sometimes after an injury, the tooth appears darker in color. Up to 70 percent of injured baby teeth darken. A dark baby tooth does not always require treatment, although these teeth are at a higher risk for dental abscess (infection). Call your child's dentist for an examination and x-ray to check for a dental abscess. The dentist can decide whether any treatment is needed.

How can teeth be damaged during a fall or accident?

Although most children escape accidents unscathed, a lot can happen to teeth during a fall. Sometimes the damage is obvious, but other times, it takes a little while to show up. Whenever your child experiences trauma to the mouth, be on the lookout for the following potential problems. If a permanent tooth is involved, be especially attentive and let your child's dentist know as soon as you notice a problem.

TOOTH HIT BUT NOT LOOSE

When teeth are hit, there may be some bleeding along the gum line without the teeth loosening. These teeth will often be sore for one to three days, but they are usually fine. Give your child a soft diet and over-the-counter pain medicine while you contact your child's dentist for an evaluation.

TOOTH HIT AND LOOSE OR OUT OF POSITION

Along with bleeding and bruising of the gum tissue, teeth may appear to be in the proper position but may wiggle back and forth or side-to-side. These teeth will often be sore for several days but will usually tighten back to normal in one or two weeks, but be sure to call your child's dentist.

Sometimes the teeth will appear slightly out of position—forward, back, extruded (high in the gum), or intruded (low). In this case, contact your child's dentist as soon as possible for evaluation. In the meantime, if the tooth is forward or back, apply firm pressure with a washcloth to try to reposition it and to control bleeding of the gum tissue. Try to minimize any more movement. Check to see if your child can close his teeth together normally. Give your child a soft diet and over-the-counter pain medications as needed, making sure he avoids chewing or biting for several days. Check whether the tooth is loose by applying gentle pressure with the tip of your fingernail. Once the tooth stabilizes, it is safe for your child to resume biting with the tooth.

TOOTH HIT AND BROKEN

It doesn't require a lot of pressure for a tooth to become chipped. Chipped teeth may be sensitive to cold and heat. Bleeding from the center or inside of the tooth indicates a fracture into the nerve of the tooth, which may be a sign of more significant damage. Contact your child's dentist as soon as possible for an evaluation and treatment recommendations.

My daughter just knocked out a permanent tooth playing baseball. What should I do?

Knocked-Out Baby Teeth

If a baby tooth is knocked out, do not attempt to reinsert the tooth into the socket because it could damage the developing adult tooth underneath. If you are at all uncertain whether the tooth is a baby tooth or permanent, place the tooth in a container of whole milk and contact your child's dentist. (It has to be whole milk, not 2% or skim.) Getting help quickly and taking care of the tooth on the way to the dentist are both important. A dentist needs to be seen within 2 hours if possible; within 30 minutes is ideal. In the meantime, you can provide over-the-counter pain medicine and a soft diet as needed. Control any bleeding with firm pressure from a cloth.

Two million teeth are knocked out each year due to all types of accidents. This happens to roughly one in every two hundred children each year. When a tooth is knocked out, the whole tooth is gone from its socket, which means it can often be replanted. Replanting a knocked-out tooth is far less expensive than replacing a missing tooth. It is also less painful and far more aesthetically pleasing.

If this happens to your child, find the tooth, handling it by the crown (or top part), not the root portion. Do not clean or handle the tooth unnecessarily. Gently rinse (but do not scrub) the tooth if possible, since you are going to want to replace it back in the socket. If your child is old enough that she won't swallow the tooth, she can "store" the tooth in her mouth, holding it in place by biting on gauze. If it is not possible for you to replace the tooth, put it in whole milk (other types of milk are too watered down to preserve the tooth as needed), a save-a-tooth solution (which many school clinics keep on hand), or even saliva. Use a soft container if possible. Avoid using glass. If the tooth is fractured, save any pieces you can find. You must get to a dentist as quickly as possible. Time is a critical factor in saving the tooth.

My son hit his tooth a few days ago, and now he is complaining of a toothache. What should I do?

Even if you don't notice anything right away, a toothache after an injury could be a sign of an infection or an abscess. Contact your child's dentist immediately. Then clean the area of the affected tooth thoroughly. Rinse the mouth vigorously with warm water and use dental floss to dislodge stuck food or debris. Never place aspirin on the gum or on the aching tooth; children should not have aspirin, due to the risk of Reye syndrome. If your child's mouth appears swollen, apply a cold compress to the outside of the mouth, protecting the skin with a towel or cloth.

> **Tooth Abscess**
>
> An abscess is a collection of pus that is caused by a bacterial infection. A tooth abscess is usually the result of an untreated cavity or a crack or chip in the tooth that allows bacteria into the inner area. To treat an abscess, the infection must be drained. Sometimes a root canal must be done to save the tooth. If the infection is serious, the tooth must be pulled. An untreated abscess can lead to life-threatening complications.

How will my daughter know if she chipped or cracked her tooth?

When a tooth chips or breaks, it may not hurt, but your child's tongue will usually feel the sharp area in a hurry. Most minor tooth fractures don't hurt, but if a large piece of the tooth breaks off, it can cause pain because the nerve inside the tooth is damaged. If it is exposed to air, or hot or cold foods or drinks, it can feel even worse.

Pain from a broken or cracked tooth may be constant or may come and go. Chewing often causes pain because it puts pressure on the tooth. There is no way to treat a cracked tooth at home. Your child needs to see a dentist. Until you get to the dentist's office, rinse your child's mouth well with warm water. Apply pressure with a piece of gauze on any bleeding areas for about 10 minutes or until the bleeding stops. Some say using a wet tea bag with pressure also helps reduce swelling and pain. If you can't get to the dentist right away, cover the sharp part of the tooth with temporary dental cement. You can find this at a drugstore. Give your child an over-the-counter pain reliever for pain if needed.

Tooth Repair

Different types of tooth fractures and breaks require different treatment, so it is always important to have your child's dentist assess the situation and the severity of the damage.

Minor cracks and chips. These only affect the surface of the tooth and rarely need treatment, but your child should see the dentist right away to assess the damage. Sometimes they feel bigger than they actually are. If there are rough spots, the dentist can lightly polish them out, returning a smooth surface to the tooth. For larger chips, your child's dentist may suggest repairing the damage with filling material to prevent it from chipping more or to make the tooth look and feel better.

Bigger cracks. These fractures involve the entire tooth, all the way down to the nerve. Although the pieces remain in place, the crack eventually spreads if not fixed. These cracks can sometimes be repaired with filling material, but a crown might be necessary to prevent the crack from getting worse and further weakening the tooth. If the crack affects the nerve, a root canal may be needed.

Broken cusp. These breaks affect only the cusp, or pointed chewing surfaces, and not the pulp. Therefore, they are unlikely to cause much pain. Your child's dentist can repair the damage and restore the tooth's shape with a crown.

Serious breaks. Some breaks go deep enough to expose the nerve, usually causing pain, sensitivity, and bleeding. If this occurs, your child will likely need root canal treatment to remove the exposed nerve and a crown to restore the tooth to normal function.

Split tooth. This means that the tooth has split vertically into two separate parts. In teeth with more than one root, it may be possible to keep one of the roots and cover it with a crown. If not, a root canal treatment or tooth extraction may be needed.

Decay-induced break. Severe cavities that weaken teeth from the inside out can cause them to break or crumble. Your child's dentist will evaluate the damage and recommend the best way to restore or remove the tooth.

Protecting Your Child's Teeth during Sports

Dental injuries are the most common type of sports injury among children. A mouth guard fits over the upper or lower teeth to prevent broken or chipped teeth from tooth-to-tooth contact. For many contact sports, like football, lacrosse, and field hockey, mouth guards are highly recommended—even if the athlete wears a helmet. A mouth guard is appropriate for "non-contact" sports as well, such as baseball, basketball, soccer, and gymnastics, where contact with solid objects and other participants is actually common. The American Dental Association estimates that mouth guards prevent approximately 200,000 injuries each year in high school and college football alone.

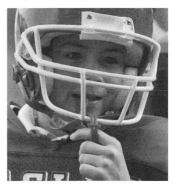

Mouth guards come in a variety of styles. © iStockphoto.com/jpbcpa

What mouth guard should my child have?

A wide range of mouth guard products are available that vary in price and the protection they offer. A properly fitted mouth guard must be protective, comfortable, resilient, tear resistant, odorless, and tasteless; it must not be bulky, and it must minimally interfere with speaking and breathing. Most important, it must have excellent retention and fit and be thick enough in critical areas.

Stock mouth guards, available at most sporting goods stores, come in three sizes (small, medium, and large) and are the least expensive (between $5 and $25) but also the least protective.

It is worth the investment to pay a little more for a boil-and-bite mouth guard. These are available in most sporting goods stores, cost about $25, and have more of a custom fit than stock guards. Hot water is used to adjust the plastic comfortably around the teeth. The difference in effectiveness between a stock mouth guard and a boil-and-bite mouth guard is substantial. Needless to say, most dentists consider the price difference well worth it.

The best option is to have your child's dentist provide a custom lab-created mouth guard built on an impression of your child's bite. It may take a week or more to create, and you'll pay more for it, but it provides several advantages:

- Clearer speech—when communication with teammates is important
- More comfortable fit—so it's less distracting
- Less restricted breathing—for improved performance

If your child plays any sports, you need to talk to his dentist about the risk for dental injuries and how to best protect his teeth. As child athletes grow, changes in their tooth position and jaw size will require changes in the mouth guard. Be sure your child visits the dentist regularly to have the fit of the mouth guard checked.

Do I have to do anything to take care of the mouth guard?

Unfortunately, mouth guards can harbor bacteria, which means they can be unhealthy (not to mention smelly). Follow these suggestions for safe mouth guard practices:

- Soak the mouth guard in an antimicrobial solution after practice or games. Keep it in the solution until it is needed again. Gently brush the mouth guard with a toothbrush periodically.
- Make sure your child avoids hanging the mouth guard on helmets, facemasks, or other dirty surfaces between plays.
- Inspect the mouth guard regularly for cracks, jagged edges, and general wear.
- Replace the mouth guard when damage or wear develops.

CHAPTER 19

Oral Surgery, Extractions, and Root Canals

The mere mention of oral surgery makes most of us shudder. Although no parents want their children to undergo oral surgery, it is sometimes necessary. In fact, almost 80 percent of people under the age of 25 need to have their wisdom teeth removed.

The good news is that, unlike other surgeries, dental surgery doesn't usually involve being admitted to a hospital or having to undergo general anesthesia. But like other types of surgery, it isn't a good idea for anyone to drive home afterward, regardless of age or driving experience. Recuperating from oral surgery can make for a rough couple of days, but many dental and oral surgery procedures—from wisdom tooth removal to implants—are less traumatic than other types of surgery.

Oral Surgery for Children

Oral and maxillofacial surgery is a specialized field of dentistry focusing on the diagnosis and surgical treatment of diseases, injuries, and birth defects that affect the jaws, mouth, gums, teeth, and facial structures. Oral maxillofacial surgeons are dental specialists whose training includes an undergraduate degree, a four-year graduate degree in dentistry, and a minimum four-year hospital surgical residency program.

Oral surgeons work as a team with orthodontists and dentists to treat children and adults who have problems with the growth and position of their jaws and teeth. One of the most common such problems in children is an adult tooth that can't come out because it's stuck in the jaw bone. The oral surgeon performs an operation so that the orthodontist can put a brace on the teeth to help pull the adult tooth down. Another common problem is when a child has too many teeth to fit in a little mouth. The orthodontist aligns the teeth properly and uses appliances that expand the inside of the mouth. Then the oral surgeon does an operation to change the bones in the jaw so that the whole mouth works properly and the child's face is balanced normally.

> *Finding an Oral Surgeon*
> Ask your child's dentist, orthodontist, and pediatrician for recommendations for an oral surgeon they trust. To find an oral and maxillofacial surgeon in your community, you can also visit the Find a Surgeon database at the American Association of Oral and Maxillofacial Surgeons at www.aaoms.org.

Some children don't have a problem with their teeth. Instead, they have difficulty related to an incorrectly developing jaw, which affects how they look, talk, and bite. Jaw problems may make it hard or painful to eat certain foods and may affect speech. To correct these problems, children's teeth are aligned by the orthodontist before the oral surgeon can perform an operation on their jaws. The orthodontist sets the stage, and the oral surgeon finishes the job. Through surgery, the jaws can be moved backward, forward, up, or down. Surgery can also change the way the bones in the face grow.

Just like the architects who plan a building, orthodontists, dentists, and oral surgeons look at the face and the jaw and try to determine the correct balance for putting the face in just the right position. They decide by taking panoramic x-rays that show the bones of the whole face and head. Information from the x-rays is transferred to a computer, and the oral surgeon uses computer software to draw different plans for correcting the problem and then chooses the best plan for making the child's face look great and function properly.

Anesthesia and Sedation

Most routine dental procedures (such as cleanings) do not require anesthesia, but some type of anesthesia is generally required for tooth extractions, root canals, fillings, and treating dental infections, such as when draining pus. In this chapter, we describe general anesthesia and sedation, but the most commonly used anesthesia for dental procedures is local anesthesia.

Local anesthesia is any technique used to remove sensation in part of the body, including the sensation of pain. Most people are comfortable with local anesthesia, which can be safely administered even in a very young child. Agreeing to the use of local anesthesia for your child is important: it reduces discomfort and keeps pain to a minimum. If your child experiences pain during a dental procedure, he will likely resist dental care in the future.

> *Information You Should Always Share with Your Child's Dentist*
>
> If you are taking your child for dental treatment under anesthesia, be sure to let the dentist know if your child has experienced
>
> jaundice or malaria in the last three months
> any liver disease
> any bleeding disorders
> any other medical treatment, including medications
> systemic disorders

When is general anesthesia recommended?

General anesthesia is a controlled state of unconsciousness that eliminates awareness, movement, and discomfort during dental treatments and other procedures. In other words, the child remains completely asleep and will not remember the procedure. This form of anesthesia may be appropriate for children who need extensive dental work or surgery; for those who have special health care needs; for those who are extremely uncooperative, fearful, or anxious; or for young children who aren't able to cooperate. Your child's dentist will discuss the benefits and risks of general anesthesia and why it is—or is not—recommended for your child.

A physician or dentist with specialized training can use various medications to provide general anesthesia for children receiving dental care. Although there is some risk associated with general anesthesia, it can usually be used safely and effectively when administered by an appropriately trained individual in an appropriately equipped facility, usually a hospital setting. Precautions are taken to protect your child during anesthesia and your child will be monitored very closely throughout the procedure to prevent any complications.

A physical evaluation by your child's primary health care provider is required prior to general anesthesia for dental care to ensure the safety of your child during the procedure. Your child's dentist or the anesthesiologist will advise you about any required pre-procedure evaluation appointments or any other necessary instructions. Parents must let the dentist know of any illness that occurs prior to the appointment, as well as medications taken, including any over-the-counter medications. For your child's safety, you may need to reschedule if she is ill or has recently been ill. It is essential to follow instructions about how long your child needs to refrain from eating or drinking before the surgical appointment.

Your child will be discharged after treatment once she is stable and alert. Often, children are still tired for several hours. You will be instructed to let your child rest at home with minimal activity until the next day. Postoperative recommendations about eating will also be given before you leave.

What is sedation dentistry?

Sedation is often used to keep children calm and comfortable before and during dental treatments. Most sedating medications work by tamping down the central nervous system. For dental treatments, sedation is given in one of three ways: through an IV, taken orally, or by inhalation (called inhalation conscious sedation).

IV sedation. Also known as moderate conscious sedation, IV sedation is usually used by oral surgeons and dentists who have specialized training and certification. With this type of sedation, medications are administered directly into the bloodstream through an IV. The greatest advantage of IV sedation is that if someone is not sedated enough, more medication can be administered and the effects are instantaneous. This method is not used in most regular dental offices because of the specialized training required and the requirements for certification by the State Board of Dentistry. The advantages of this approach are that the drugs used for IV sedation are more effective than the same drugs taken orally, and children have less memory of the procedure with this technique than with others.

Orally administered sedation. In this sedation, the child takes a pill or liquid medication. All body functions remain normal, and she is able to breathe on her own. Although patients remain conscious, many relax so deeply that they fall asleep. Some degree of amnesia is common. For children, the most common medication used is midazolam (Versed), which is a liquid. The disadvantage with this method of sedation is that it is impossible to predict how a child will respond to the medication.

Inhalation conscious sedation. Nitrous oxide/oxygen sedation, also known as laughing gas, is the most frequently used sedation method in dentistry. All body functions remain normal, and the child is able to breathe on her own. Many children fall asleep and experience some degree of amnesia about what happened during their dental appointment. Inhalation sedation has been used by dentists for many years.

My dentist said she wants to use conscious sedation. What does that mean?

This concept in pediatric dentistry may be new to most parents. Sedation dentistry, sometimes called relaxation dentistry, refers to how dentists manage pain and anxiety during dental appointments. Conscious sedation typically means a minimally depressed level of consciousness, where patients are able to respond to commands and breathe on their own. During interactive conscious sedation, a child can respond to verbal requests from the dentist and keep his eyes open, even while being sedated.

Although most children are cooperative during dental treatment, some have difficulty, especially young or fearful children. These children may benefit from behavior management techniques discussed elsewhere in this book, such as good communication—including controlling your tone of voice; the Tell, Show, Do method; reassuring nonverbal communication; and positive reinforcement—as well as using distraction and deciding whether it's better for the parent to be present or absent during the procedure. If these behavior management techniques don't work, conscious sedation can help. Your child's dentist will always ask for your written consent before attempting conscious sedation. You should understand any procedure completely before agreeing to it, including sedation.

During the procedure, even though your child is sedated,

- he is not unconscious
- his reflexes (ability to react) are absolutely normal
- his breathing is continuous, spontaneous, and unobstructed
- he can respond to all kinds of physical stimuli and verbal commands

If your child is to be given conscious sedation,

- provide the anesthesiologist or dentist with accurate medical history and information about any allergies your child has
- learn about the side effects
- carefully follow the list of instructions given by the anesthesiologist or dentist after the procedure

Tooth Extractions

Primary, or baby, teeth are important in a child's development, so every effort is made not to remove them. But one or more baby teeth may need to be removed due to decay, disease, or trauma. If so, your child's dentist can recommend a device to maintain the space until the permanent teeth come in.

Secondary, or permanent, teeth may be removed due to disease or to correct severe overcrowding. Make sure you understand the reason for the extraction. If you have any questions or concerns, you should feel free to raise them with your child's dentist. Keep asking until you are satisfied with your decision. You may decide to seek a second opinion.

How can I prepare my child to have a tooth removed?

If your child is not frightened of the dentist or the procedure, she is more likely to be excited about her upcoming tooth fairy visit than to be worried about the pain. We suggest having the tooth fairy give an extra big surprise for pulled teeth. Every child is different; talk to the dentist beforehand so you know what to say to your child and how to say it to minimize anxiety or other problems.

How is the tooth extracted?

After applying a numbing agent, the dentist will expand the tooth's socket and separate the ligaments using use a tool called an elevator, which wedges between the tooth and the bone surrounding it. Next, the extraction forceps will be used to manipulate the tooth from side to side, rotating it for further socket expansion and ligament separation. Finally, the tooth will be pulled until it completely slides out of the socket.

Does my child need special care after the extraction?

Bleeding is normal after a tooth has been extracted, lasting up to a day. After the procedure, a small piece of gauze will be applied to the area where the tooth was removed and should be kept in place long enough for the blood to clot, usually about 30 minutes. To keep your child's mouth as clean as possible during this healing period, rinse his mouth with saltwater several times per day.

Be sure to have children's acetaminophen or ibuprofen on hand in case your child's dentist does not prescribe a painkiller. A bag of ice applied to the outside of your child's jaw will help keep swelling to a minimum and may help relieve any pain. If the swelling doesn't go down or seems excessive, or if your child begins to feel ill or develops a fever, call the dentist immediately. These may be signs of an infection, which happens rarely.

Our dentist says my son has an extra tooth that needs to be removed. How is this possible?

Extra teeth are called supernumary. The most common supernumary teeth are called mesiodens, which are located in the midline of the mouth. Extra teeth can be well formed or look like little lumps of tooth-like material. They are often discovered during routine x-rays.

If the tooth interferes with the normal eruption of other teeth or if it may complicate braces, it will need to be addressed. Usually, if it's not causing an immediate problem, it can be monitored until something needs to be done. Rarely, it will erupt on its own and can be extracted. Most often, it will need to be surgically removed. It is important not to do it too soon, however, because the removal might damage the developing teeth. Sometimes 3-D x-rays are recommended to determine the correct surgical path to get it out. Fortunately, this type of oral surgery is generally straightforward, and children recover within a few days.

What is an impacted tooth?

An impacted tooth is one that is stuck or is blocked in the gums and cannot make its way into the mouth. Although we usually hear about wisdom teeth being impacted, just about any tooth can become stuck. Eyeteeth (canine teeth) often become impacted. These are usually the last of the

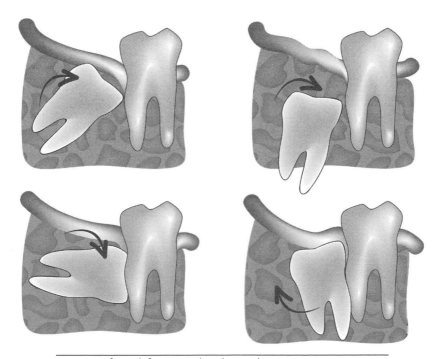

Directions of growth for impacted wisdom teeth. © Can Stock Photo Inc. / natsuk

front teeth to emerge, so space might not be available for them. Impacted teeth are usually identified during routine dental exams and x-rays.

You and your child's dentist need to talk about how to address any impacted teeth. If your child is young and still developing, sometimes the dentist can create space, encouraging the tooth to come in correctly, or use other nonsurgical techniques to uncover the impacted tooth. Other times, and often with wisdom teeth, oral surgery is recommended.

Untreated impacted teeth can be painful and lead to infection. They may also crowd or damage adjacent teeth or roots. A more serious problem occurs if the sac surrounding the impacted tooth becomes filled with fluid and enlarges to form a cyst. As the cyst grows, it may hollow out the jaw and permanently damage other teeth, the surrounding bone, and nerves. Rarely, if a cyst is not treated, a tumor may develop from its walls, and a more serious surgical procedure may be required to remove it.

What are wisdom teeth, and when are they a problem?

Wisdom teeth, also known as third molars, are the last teeth to appear. They generally erupt between the ages of 17 and 25, a time of life that has been called the "age of wisdom."

Anthropologists have noted that the rough diet of early humans resulted in excessive wear on their teeth. Normal shifting of the teeth compensated for this wear, ensuring that space was available for most wisdom teeth to erupt by adolescence with no problems. Today's much softer diet, along

> *Does Everyone Have Wisdom Teeth?*
>
> No. Between 25 and 30 percent of people do not have all four wisdom teeth. They might have just three, two, one, or none.

with the common use of braces, produces a fuller dental arch, not leaving enough room for the wisdom teeth to erupt. This can cause problems when the final four molars come in.

Do wisdom teeth have to come out if they aren't hurting?

Not all problems related to wisdom teeth are painful or visible. In fact, damage can occur without your being aware of it. As wisdom teeth grow, their roots become longer and stronger, making the tooth more difficult to remove. Impacted wisdom teeth that are left in are more likely to cause problems as a person ages. Third molars that have broken through the tissue and erupted into the mouth partially or in a normal upright position may be just as prone to disease as any wisdom teeth that remain impacted. It is hard to brush that far back in the mouth, so bits of food and bacteria get stuck, which can cause infections, gum disease, and pain. No one can predict when complications with wisdom teeth will occur. All of this adds up to one answer: in most cases, wisdom teeth need to come out before any problems arise.

When should wisdom teeth be removed?

It isn't wise to wait until wisdom teeth start to bother your child. In general, earlier removal of wisdom teeth results in a less complicated procedure and healing process. Ideally, wisdom teeth should be removed by the time your child is a young adult, to prevent future problems and to ensure optimal healing. If the wisdom teeth remain, your child may be at greater risk for damaged teeth and disease, including periodon-

> *Plan Ahead for TLC*
>
> Prepare for recuperation before you take your child to have the procedure done. Stock the freezer with Popsicles and ice packs, create a nesting spot in a semi-reclined chair, and pick up pain relievers before the surgery so that you can bring your child straight home and into a comfy spot.

titis (gum disease), in the tissues surrounding the third molars and adjacent teeth, and these gum infections can harm a person's general health as he gets older. If you decide not to remove them or want to delay the surgery, talk to your child's dentist about appropriate care and follow-up in order to prevent any complications.

What happens during wisdom teeth surgery?

How easy it is to remove a wisdom tooth depends on several conditions, including the position of the tooth and the tooth's root development. Impacted wisdom teeth may require a more involved surgical procedure. Before surgery, your child's oral and maxillofacial surgeon will talk with you and your child about what to expect. Ask any questions you have and express any concerns. As with all surgeries, it is important to let the doctor know about any illness your child has and medications she is taking.

Most wisdom tooth extractions are performed in the oral surgeon's office under local anesthesia, intravenous sedation, or general anesthesia. Your child's surgeon will discuss all the details of the anesthetic options with you and choose one that's right for your child. After surgery, your child will experience some swelling and mild discomfort. These reactions are part of the normal healing process. Cold compresses on the outside of the mouth may help decrease the swelling, and medication prescribed by the surgeon can help manage the discomfort. You may be instructed to modify your child's diet after surgery and gradually progress to more normal foods. Expect the healing process to take several days. Many families schedule the procedure over summer vacation or during another extended break from school.

> *Oral Contraceptive May Increase Pain after Wisdom Tooth Extraction*
>
> An 2003 article in the *British Dental Journal* suggested that young women taking birth control pills are more susceptible than young women not taking the pill to both postoperative pain and dry socket (infection of the socket). The reason isn't fully known. The pill may reduce the pain threshold so that the woman feels more pain. Talk to your oral surgeon about any medication your child is on.

How can I prevent dry socket after my child's teeth are removed?

Alveolar osteitis, commonly called dry socket, is a condition that affects many people who undergo tooth extraction. The socket is the hole in the bone where the tooth has been removed. After a tooth is removed, a blood clot forms in the socket to protect the bone and the nerves underneath. Sometimes that clot becomes dislodged or dissolves after the extraction. That leaves the bone and nerve exposed to air, food, fluid, and anything else that enters the mouth. This can lead to infection and severe pain that can last up to a week. Pain from dry socket typically starts about two days after the tooth was pulled. Over time it becomes more severe and can radiate to the ear.

Some people are more likely to get dry socket, including those who smoke, have poor oral hygiene, or use birth control pills. Dry sockets are also more common with traumatic extractions or unusually long procedures. Drinking through a straw after having a tooth extracted can also increase the risk of getting dry socket. Your child should try not to rinse her mouth or disturb the socket area for the first day.

If you suspect that your child has a dry socket, look into the site where the tooth was pulled. You should see a blood clot, not just bone. Other symptoms of dry socket include bad breath and an unpleasant taste in the mouth. Your child's dentist or oral surgeon will manage the dry socket by cleaning the tooth socket, removing any debris from the hole, and then filling the socket with a medicated piece of gauze or a special paste to promote healing.

Expect to take your child back to the office every day for a dressing change until the socket starts to heal and the pain lessens. Antibiotics may be prescribed to prevent the socket from becoming infected. If a nonsteroidal anti-inflammatory drug (NSAID) such as ibuprofen doesn't ease the discomfort, let the dentist or doctor know, so that a stronger pain medication can be prescribed.

> *Caring for Dry Sockets*
>
> If your child develops a dry socket, she can relieve pain and keep the healing on track by following these guidelines:
>
> - Hold cold packs to the outside of your face to help decrease pain and swelling.
> - Take pain medications as prescribed.
> - Avoid smoking or using tobacco products.
> - Drink plenty of clear liquids to remain hydrated and to prevent nausea that may be associated with some pain medications.
> - Rinse your mouth gently with warm salt water several times a day.
> - Brush your teeth gently around the dry socket area.

Root Canals

A root canal is sometimes needed to repair and save a tooth that is badly decayed or infected. If a root canal is needed, your child's dentist might refer you to an endodontist, a dental specialist who performs root canals.

A root canal is the term used to describe the natural cavity within the center of the tooth. The pulp of the tooth is the hollow inner core within the root canal. The pulp contains nerves, blood vessels, connective tissue, and reparative cells (which take part in healing). Pulp therapy involves treating problems with this part of the tooth. A cavity that involves the nerve (pulp) of the tooth may cause intense pain. Although the pain may subside for a time if your child takes ibuprofen or antibiotics, it will return unless the tooth is properly treated. When the nerve of the tooth is infected, it must be treated to restore good dental health.

A pediatric root canal procedure is referred to as a pulpotomy, or a baby or children's root canal. A pulpotomy is performed when the decay in a child's tooth reaches the pulp and affects the nerves. The infected part of the nerve within the crown portion of the tooth is removed to prevent further inflammation and spread of disease. The canals are cleansed and disinfected. After a root canal, the teeth are filled with a special material before the outside is restored. If the tooth is a back molar, it is restored with a stainless steel crown to re-establish normal chewing function. For a primary tooth, this crown continues to hold the space until the permanent tooth can take its place. On the upper front teeth, either a stainless steel or tooth-colored crown can be placed. This procedure is performed in one visit and causes no more discomfort than a routine filling.

I've always heard root canals are no fun. How can I prepare my child?

Root canals are usually dreaded by adults who, too often, share their feelings about the procedure with their child. Imagine a child's anxiety when faced with this procedure after being forewarned by her parents. Parents can prepare their children and calm their fears a great deal simply by watching how they talk about the procedure. For most people, root canals are not that bad. In fact, many say that having a root canal is similar to having a deep filling. Dental procedures and pain management techniques have greatly improved. Your child, who really needs the procedure, is already hurting. After the root canal, he will feel much better than he does right now. Focus on the here and now and don't ratchct up your child's stress level because of your own experience or what you've heard from others.

Dental Implants in Children

It's every parent's fear—a child losing a permanent tooth due to a sports injury or other mishap, especially if there's a big gap when the child smiles. According to some dentists, the solution is a dental implant: an artificial tooth root that resembles a golf tee, which supports an artificial tooth (or teeth). Although implants were initially developed as an alternative treatment to removable dentures, they have been used successfully in children for about a decade.

The timing of implant surgery in children is critical, however, since children's jaws are still growing. With growth, there is the possibility that the implant can gradually sink into the bone. In general, dental implants can be done any time after adolescence or when bone growth is complete. Although the optimal timing of implants remains unclear, most dental experts agree that it's best to wait until after the jaw has matured, usually by age 17 or 18 for girls and 19 or 20 for boys.

A dental implant is a specialized and involved procedure requiring several consultations beforehand as well as follow-up during the recovery and aftercare. Prep time is needed beforehand to make sure there is enough bone in three dimensions to support the implant. Additionally, many dentists recommend a cone CT scan in advance. The implant procedure itself takes approximately 15 to 20 minutes per implant after the anesthesia kicks in.

Dental implants are made of titanium (the same material in artificial hips), a highly biocompatible metal that bone grows into via a process known as osseointegration. (Biocompatible means that the material is compatible with the human body and is unlikely to be rejected by the body.) In the past, it took up to six months for the bone to integrate with the implant. However, surface changes made in the metal now speed the process, and integration takes only two or three months. Manufacturers etch the surface of the implants, creating microscopic pits and valleys. Bone cells fill the pits and valleys, forming a strong bond. Once integrated, implants stimulate bone growth. An integrated implant is much stronger than a natural tooth.

Implants can fail if they do not anchor to the jawbone. Even though most patients receive antibiotics following the surgery, infections still sometimes occur.

Preparation and Aftercare for Oral Surgery

Consult with your child's oral surgeon or dentist before the oral surgery to find out what to expect. Discuss any concerns or fears you have. Your child's dentist will be more than happy to discuss sedation options and distraction methods that may help your child through the oral surgery. If your child will require any medications after the procedure, especially for pain relief, prepare ahead so that you can have them ready.

If your child's dentist or oral surgeon is using intravenous sedation or general anesthetic, follow all preoperative instructions closely. Generally, your child should not eat or drink anything, including water, for 8 hours before the oral surgery. If your child's surgery requires local anesthetic, she can have a light meal 1 to 2 hours before the procedure. Make sure she brushes and flosses her teeth prior to the appointment.

Your child should wear short-sleeved, loose-fitting, comfortable clothing for the appointment. Although the doctor and staff do their best to prevent staining garments, she should wear something she won't mind getting stained. Your child should not wear jewelry to the appointment because it must be removed before some procedures. If she wears glasses or contact lenses, she'll need to remove them before the procedure. She should also avoid makeup, although you can bring along some lip balm because her lips may become chapped during the surgery.

What are the potential complications of oral surgery or more complex dental procedures?

BLEEDING

Bleeding is the most common problem following oral surgery. The best treatment for bleeding is constant, firm pressure applied to the bleeding area using gauze packs. Place the packs so that when your child closes his mouth, pressure is applied to the area. Hold gauze pressure for 20 minutes, then change the gauze or remove it, if bleeding has stopped. The only substitute for gauze is a moist tea bag, held over the area for 60 minutes. If profuse bleeding continues, call the office. Your child should not use mouthwash for the first 24 hours after surgery. Vigorous rinsing during this time will increase bleeding.

SWELLING

Oral surgical procedures are usually followed by some swelling, which will be more noticeable on the second and third day. For the first 24 hours after surgery, keep your child's head above his heart (semi-reclined) and apply ice bags over the area of the surgery. After 24 hours, it should not be necessary to continue with cold applications.

The day after the procedure, saltwater mouth rinses (½ teaspoon of salt to a cup of warm water) every 2 to 3 hours (six times per day) may help reduce the swelling and postoperative pain. The temperature of the water should be as warm as possible without causing any damage from burning. Your child should continue to use the saltwater rinses for the next 14 days. A solution of half hydrogen peroxide and half water can also be used once a day to speed healing and protect against infection. The swelling will usually last for 10 days to 2 weeks and be accompanied by a fever of 99 to 101 degrees F.

JAW STIFFNESS

Jaw stiffness is due to a tightening of the muscles of the jaw. This stiffness makes it difficult to open the mouth for a few days to weeks. To prevent stiffness and to stimulate circulation, a gentle daily program to exercise the muscles, such as by chewing gum, will help.

BONY FRAGMENTS

During the healing process, small, sharp fragments of bone may loosen and work up through the gum. Since they do not contain roots, they often work their way out themselves. If not, your child should return to the dentist to have them removed through a simple procedure.

DISCOLORATION

After surgery in the mouth, the soft tissues have been replaced and sutured in position. In some cases, there is initial bleeding beneath the tissues. Discoloration will follow and is perfectly normal. Heat in any form will help it disappear.

PAIN

Surgical operations in the highly sensitive oral cavity can be expected to produce some postoperative pain. If a pain prescription has been given, your child should take the medication only as needed. Occasionally, severe pain will develop in the jaw, face, or ear, from two days to two weeks after surgery. The pain is sometimes accompanied by a bad taste in the mouth. In most cases, this indicates that the blood clot in the tooth socket has decomposed, exposing the bony walls of the socket in a condition called dry socket, or alveolar osteitis (see above). If these symptoms occur, call the dental office to return for a checkup.

What can my daughter eat after surgery?

Diet after oral surgery generally consists of soft foods that require little or no chewing. Your child should avoid food that is spicy or acidic, because they may irritate the gum tissue. Beverages that contain a high nutritional value, such as Boost, Slim Fast, Ensure, or protein powder shake mixes, are easy to prepare and provide much of the vitamins and minerals necessary to stay nourished during recovery. Do not let your child use a straw, especially after a tooth extraction. Sucking on a straw can cause dry socket (see above), which requires additional treatment from the dentist.

Is it okay to brush after surgery?

Yes. Your child should brush her teeth three times a day, avoiding the surgical site, and clean her gums using saltwater on a cotton applicator. She may also speed healing and eliminate complications by keeping her mouth clean with gentle rinsing and being careful to avoid injury and irritation to the surgical area. After every solid food meal, she should continue using saltwater rinses for 14 days after surgery.

What can I do to keep my son comfortable?

Prepare your child's bed and living space comfortably, so he can get the rest he needs after oral surgery. Use pillows to keep him semi-reclined, because he most likely will not be able to sleep flat on his back or on his side. Be sure to use an old pillowcase and sheet set in case of stains from bleeding. Keep books, word puzzles, and magazines within easy reach of the resting area to help pass the time. If he enjoys watching television shows, movies, or playing video games, relocate your television set, if possible, into the room where he will be spending the most time recovering.

CHAPTER 20 ▼

Dental Anxiety

Many people experience severe fears that lead them to avoid the feared situation, object, or activity. Some of these fears might seem irrational to other people, but they can cause great distress and can influence other aspects of a person's life. Dental fear is the term used to describe many types of dental fears and anxieties—some rational, some seemingly irrational. Anxiety in general is extremely common, and most people experience some degree of dental anxiety, especially if they are about to have something done that they have never had done before. This is fear of the unknown. Other fears are reactions to a known danger, including awareness of what the dentist is going to do, because the person has been to the dentist before and had it done. "Been there, done that—and I'm scared!"

Dental Fear

Anyone can experience dental fear. It doesn't matter who you are—young or old, male or female, rich or poor. The good news is that helping your child open up about her fears can lift a huge weight off her shoulders. Dentists are used to people who are anxious or phobic. It is common to be at least a little afraid of the dentist. Encourage your child to be honest with her dentist and not try to hide her fear or anxiety.

Why is being afraid of the dentist such a big deal?

Dental fears can have significant consequences for life. Not only is a person's dental health likely to suffer, he is prone to anxiety and depression if he has poorly cared for teeth. Depending on how obvious the damage is, embarrassment about his teeth can lead the person to avoid meeting people, even close friends, as well as situations that involve contact with the public. Loss of self-esteem over not being able to do something as simple as going to a dentist as well as intense feelings of guilt about not taking care of one's teeth properly are also very common.

What are the most common causes of dental fears?

Dental fears are most often caused by bad or, in some cases, horrific experiences at a dentist's office. The experiences may have involved pain or feeling embarrassed. Maybe the dentist or hygienist made insensitive, mean, or humiliating remarks. In fact, intense feelings of shame and embarrassment are a main contributor to dental fears. Human beings are social animals, and negative social evaluation upsets all but the most thick-skinned individuals. If you're a sensitive person, negative feedback can be shattering.

Dental fears are also common in people who have been abused. A history of being bullied or physically or emotionally abused by a person in authority may also contribute to developing dental fears, especially in combination with bad experiences with dentists.

It is often thought, even among dental professionals, that the fear of pain keeps people from seeing a dentist. However, this avoidance usually has more to do with the attitude and personality of the dentist and dental staff. Pain caused by a dentist who is perceived as cold and controlling can have a huge psychological effect, while pain caused by a dentist who is perceived as caring is much less likely to result in psychological trauma.

Another cause of dental fear is observational learning. If a parent or other caregiver is afraid of dentists, children may pick up on their fear and learn to be afraid as well, even if they don't personally have bad experiences. Hearing other people's horror stories can have a similar effect. Also, the depiction of "the dentist" in the media, particularly in cartoons and children's movies, can cause children to develop dental fears.

To avoid having your child pick up on your dental fear, you will need to address your own anxiety. If you've had bad experiences with dentists in the past, it is easy to make the assumption that all dentists are uncaring or unkind. Even if you've had the misfortune of running into more than one unkind dentist, this does not mean that *all* dentists are unkind. It simply means that you were unlucky in the past. Fortunately, there are a lot of caring and gentle dentists around—for you and for your child.

What is a dental phobia?

Few people look forward to visiting the dentist, but for an estimated 7 to 13 percent of the population, the feeling is much stronger. They have a dentophobia—literally, "dental phobia"—which can prevent them from getting even regular checkups. A person with a phobia may think, "I know what happens when I go to the dentist. There's no way I'm going back if I can help it. I'm so terrified, I feel sick." The fight-or-flight response can be conjured up just thinking about or being reminded of the threatening situation. Someone with a dental phobia will avoid dental care at all costs until severe pain or a major problem gives them no choice.

It's not easy to define dental phobia, because dental fear may feel just as frightening as a real phobia. Many people view themselves as having a phobia when they really have fear. The term dental phobia is often used for any feeling of terror at the thought of dentists or dentistry or even anything dental related. Some people feel that their fear is justified and rational, while others feel silly or embarrassed for getting so upset about something that everyone else considers normal and routine.

Preventing and Managing Dental Fears

The first step in overcoming fear of the dentist is to gather accurate information. Knowledge is a powerful weapon against fear. In fact, many people's dental anxieties are just fears of the great unknown. Being afraid of pain or injury is even a good thing to a degree. It prevents us from hurting ourselves and keeps us safe. It is not surprising, then, that when we are faced with a situation we think will be painful, we try to avoid it, which unfortunately leads some people to avoid dental care and endure years of discomfort from their teeth. Once you and your child develop trust with the dentist, dental fears quickly evaporate. Going to the dentist is not nearly as bad as living each day with bad teeth.

What if I'm afraid my dentist will scold me about my child's oral health?

Many parents fear being chastised by the dentist for neglecting their child's mouth and not coming to the dentist sooner or more often. They might expect the dentist to reprimand them like a disapproving parent or schoolteacher. While some dentists used to think it was helpful to lecture patients about what they were doing wrong or to teach them a lesson, most dentists today realize that instead of being helpful, this approach often drives people away or makes them dislike the dentist. What's important is that the person is coming in for dental care *now*. Nothing you have done will shock the dentist, and plenty of dentists truly care about helping their patients no matter who they are or what they have done (or not done) in the past. They are just happy you came in.

Many people complain that their dentists never explain to them what they are doing to their mouth and why. Instead of being treated like a whole person, people feel like the dentist is only interested in their teeth. Today, most dentists view their patients as partners. Everyone must work together to ensure good dental care. Any treatments that are being suggested, how procedures are done, what they involve from the patient's point of view, what the alternatives are, and what the pros and cons of the various options are must be explained to you in detail by your child's dentist. If they aren't, be sure to speak up and ask. With children, parents must give informed consent before any treatment is started. Nothing should be done to your child's teeth without your knowing what the procedure is and agreeing to it. Don't ever feel pressured to make a decision right away if you aren't ready. If you need to take some time to think about it or talk with others, it's okay.

I hate not knowing what the dentist is doing in my child's mouth. What should I do to make myself and my child feel more comfortable?

Before your child undergoes any procedure, ask the dentist about what will be done, what sensations your child can expect to feel next, what types of noises she will hear, and so on. Most dentists love talking about teeth and are more than happy to explain their work to you. They can even show you what tools they are going to use (and some of them are quite interesting, especially to children) and demonstrate them beforehand if you like. This technique is commonly known as Tell, Show, Do. Many people who fear the loss of control like being informed in this way. It removes the element of unpredictability that many of us dread, adults and children alike.

If you or your child becomes too anxious and wants a break from the treatment, you can work with your child's dentist to establish a stop signal. Basically, this signal means "I need a break" or "I'm uncomfortable" or "I'm feeling pain." One example is raising your arm or leg. It also helps if your child's dentist takes frequent breaks during a procedure, especially at the start. This might mean that the dentist stops every few seconds and asks if you and your child are doing okay until you both feel comfortable with a procedure.

A Parent's Role in Allaying Fears

- Stress to your child how important it is to take care of your teeth and gums, including going to the dentist regularly.
- Answer all questions with simple and to-the-point answers. Don't provide any more detail than necessary. Let the dental staff provide more complex information since they are trained to describe things to children using nonthreatening and easy-to-understand language.
- Don't tell your child that it will hurt.
- Don't share your own unpleasant dental experiences.
- Stay close to your child during the dental appointment and encourage him to identify his fears out loud so that you and your child's dentist can help him remain comfortable and cooperative.

Dentist's offices are full of strange sights, sounds, and smells.
How can I help my child not be afraid?

If you or your child suffers with dental fears, merely thinking about the images, sounds, and smells associated with dentistry is enough to generate intense feelings, even panic. Some dental practice layouts, equipment, and color schemes are much friendlier than others. Does the place look clean but not too clinical or sterile? Is there a happy atmosphere or at least not a scary one? What's the overall feel of the place? If the physical environment is important to you, check out a few different practices by taking a tour of the premises or looking at pictures on their Web sites. It's amazing to see the differences between offices—some have a homey, living room–like atmosphere, while others can look downright gloomy.

You might remember from your childhood when all instruments were laid out in plain view on a tray right next to the dental chair. Today your child probably won't have to face such a view. The main reason for this is that modern standards of infection control don't allow it, but it also helps adults and children feel more at ease not having these instruments staring them directly in the face. Still, many people are scared of the sight of instruments being put into their mouths.

The reality is that dentists work in such a way that you can't really see the tools in your direct line of vision. Of course, your child may wish to see them beforehand and have them demonstrated to her. For many children, having a better look at the drill and having it demonstrated on their finger takes a lot of the fear away. They might even like to see exactly what is going on, which the dentist might be able to arrange with the help of mirrors. On the other hand, for some children, simply closing their eyes works best for them while receiving dental care.

Many people equate the sound of the drill with pain. Just hearing it may evoke a perception of pain. This is understandable if you've had a painful dentistry experience in the past that was accompanied by the sound of the tool. Although no one really enjoys the sounds at the dentist, dental drills are not as noisy as you may remember them. Also bear in mind that when noise is inserted into your mouth, it sounds much louder. This is another reason you might ask your child's dentist to demonstrate any instrument that makes a noise before it is used. Your child might want to sit up while watching the demonstration. Sitting up makes it much easier to feel in control. Many people find that their mind has been playing tricks on them, and the reality is nothing like they had imagined.

Is there such a thing as painless dentistry?

Some dental treatments can be somewhat painful on rare occasions, but most of the time, dental treatments are either completely painless or only mildly uncomfortable. Most dentists understand how pain affects their patients. They are also well aware that causing pain during treatment is no way to build a dental practice.

Dentists have many ways of reducing pain and discomfort during dental treatments. Various procedures can be done comfortably without anesthesia. If a local anesthetic is needed, strong topical anesthetic gels or patches are used to greatly reduce the discomfort of the injections. Dentists are then careful to make sure the patient's mouth is as numb as possible during treatment. This is done by approaching the treatment location slowly, constantly asking the patient how much he can feel. It takes a little longer for some people's mouths to become numb.

Any time your child feels pain, she should let the dentist know immediately. There may be some degree of pain even after everything feels numb. This can be caused by inaccurate placement of the anesthetic or not enough time allowed for it to work. The dentist can easily fix these situations by redirecting or giving more of the anesthetic or waiting longer before beginning treatment. Another important consideration is that

---

How to Talk to Your Child's Dentist

It's important to maintain an honest and open relationship with your child's dentist. Whenever any new treatments are recommended, start with these questions so there are no surprises later.

- If it was your child's tooth or mouth, what would you do?
- What does the treatment involve? How is it done? What will it feel like?
- Are there any alternatives? If so, what are the alternatives? What are the pros and cons of these alternatives?
- What will happen if I do nothing?
- How much will this treatment or procedure cost?

different people have different thresholds for pain. What hurts one person might not hurt another.

Some dental procedures, such as dental extractions, root canals, gum surgery, or multiple dental fillings, can be uncomfortable after the anesthesia has worn off. This causes many people to be concerned about pain later. Dentists are just as concerned about minimizing pain after a procedure as they are during it. They can use anesthesia that lasts longer or give additional pain medication before some procedures. Dentists are also licensed to prescribe potent drugs that are highly effective in reducing or eliminating any discomfort after dental treatments. Your child's dentist may even call you at home after a potentially painful treatment to see how things are going. Remember dentists are just as concerned as you are in relieving your child's pain and making her as comfortable as possible.

Fear of Needles

No one likes the sight of needles. It is relatively easy to distract children for the short time it takes to give an injection. These distractions can involve telling a story, petting a stuffed animal, watching a video, or giving a soothing touch. Closing their eyes can be helpful too. If your child has a severe needle phobia, talk to his dentist about psychological and pharmacological methods that might make the injection more manageable and the dental procedure a more pleasant experience.

What else can I do to help my child overcome dental fears?

TEACH YOUR CHILD RELAXATION TECHNIQUES

They are easy to learn and provide a good lifelong tool that your child can use whenever he is in a stressful or uncomfortable situation.

- *Guided imagery.* This is a simple mental technique where your child imagines having a pleasant experience or being in a soothing place. The idea is for her to create as much mental detail as she possibly can. She may become so involved in the mental images that she hardly notices what the dentist is doing.
- *Deep breathing.* Breathing slowly and deeply floods the body with oxygen and other chemicals that relax the central nervous system and help reduce discomfort.

• *Progressive relaxation.* With this technique, your child consciously tries to relax each muscle in her body, starting with the toes and moving all the way up to the head (or in reverse). Progressive relaxation reduces muscular tension while also giving you something else to think about, which can help reduce the perception of pain.

SCHEDULE SOMETHING FUN FOR AFTER YOUR CHILD'S APPOINTMENT

A visit to the park or the movies, or even puppy-gazing at the pet shop can all be fun for kids. If your child has something to look forward to while he is sitting in the dental chair, he can focus less on the appointment and more on what he will do afterward. This can make the appointment seem less like the Big Horrible Thing in his day and more like a quick errand.

BRING AN IPOD

If you give your child something else to concentrate on, this may help him relax and pay less attention to what is going on in the dental chair. Lots of dentists have televisions and music playing in the treatment rooms, but feel free to take your own iPod (with noise-reducing headphones, if those help) into the treatment room for your child. Whether it's a pop song or a fun audiobook, soothing sounds can help keep little minds off what's going on in their mouths. If all else fails, you can sing your child's favorite song to him or tell him a good story. If old enough, your child can do this for himself, silently in his head, a good lifelong skill for him to learn.

DON'T ARRIVE TOO EARLY

Nobody likes late patients, but coming to the appointment too early just means more time in the waiting room. If you or your child has dental fears, spending too much time in the waiting room before the appointment can heighten anxiety. Show up exactly on time for your child's appointment to minimize the time you have to wait. If the office staff

---

There's an App for That

British hypnotherapist, James Holmes has developed a smart phone application called Dental Phobia that provides a combination of hypnosis, relaxation techniques, and dental phobia tips to help people overcome their fear of the dentist. It's supposed to help you prepare for, and relax during, your appointment.

knows you're combating dental phobia, they may be able to whisk your child right from the front door to a treatment room or schedule her during a less busy time so that they can give her the extra attention and privacy she needs.

When It's Just Not Going to Work

Sometimes, no matter what you try, your child is just not going to sit through the dental appointment. Don't make children endure treatment if they are upset or panicked. In an emergency, it might be necessary, but generally, forcing a hysterical child to have dental treatment (even a simple cleaning) is going to backfire—no matter what. A slow, gentle approach where your child feels in charge is best. This can build her confidence and make her feel proud about overcoming her fears. But if this isn't working (at least not this time), don't stress. You can always return at another time for more treatment as necessary, especially after you have had time to think about a new plan of action.

As many of us know, bad memories of the dentist can influence how we feel about going to the dentist for the rest of our lives. Dentists know this too and are usually willing to work with you to figure out how best to get your child the dental care she needs. Just don't ever give up! Good oral health for children is too important.

> *You Know Your Child Best*
>
> Some parents say that their child does better when he doesn't even know he is off to visit the dentist until arriving at the dental office. You know your child best and what works best for him. If whatever you are doing seems to be working in getting your child to the dentist, stick with it. If not, it might be helpful to try some other tactics. The overall goal is to maintain good oral health for your child. Use whatever methods help you achieve that goal.

APPENDIX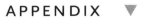

My Child's Dental Health Record

Child's Name:	
Dentist's Name:	
Address:	
Phone Number:	
Emergency Number:	
E-mail Address:	
Orthodontist's Name:	
Address:	
Phone Number:	
Emergency Number:	
E-mail Address:	

Dental Appointments

Date	Dentist's Name	Lost Tooth?	*Results*

GLOSSARY

Amalgam A silver filling.

Attrition The normal wearing down of the surface of a tooth from chewing.

Bicuspids (premolars) Teeth with two rounded points located between the eyeteeth (cuspids) and the molars.

Biofilm A thin layer of microorganisms that attaches to a surface.

Bleaching A technique that lightens the color of heavily stained teeth.

Bonding A technique to bind a filling or filling material to a tooth. Bonding materials may be used to repair chipped, cracked, misshapen, or discolored teeth or to fill in a gap between teeth.

Bridges Nonremovable tooth replacements attached to adjoining natural teeth when one or a few teeth are missing.

Bruxism Involuntary clenching or grinding of the teeth.

Calculus (tartar) Forms when dental plaque on the teeth is not removed and it hardens.

Caries The disease or process that causes tooth decay.

Cast restoration A procedure that uses a model of the tooth to make a casting that replaces missing parts.

Cementum The bonelike tissue that covers the root of the tooth.

Centrals (laterals) The four front teeth.

Crown (cap) The artificial covering of a tooth with metal, porcelain, or porcelain fused to metal. Crowns cover teeth weakened by decay or severely damaged or chipped.

Cusp The pointed or rounded part of a tooth's biting surface.

Cuspids The teeth near the front of the mouth that come to a single point. Sometimes called the eyeteeth or canines.

Dentin The layer of tooth underneath the enamel that composes the main part of the tooth.

Dentofacial orthopedics A branch of dentistry that treats abnormal tooth and jaw relationships.

Enamel The hard white surface that covers the crown of a tooth.

Endodontics Treatment of the root and nerve of the tooth.

Eruption When a new tooth becomes visible in the mouth, "erupting" through the gums.

Gingivitis An inflammation of the gums surrounding the teeth caused by a buildup of plaque, tartar, or food particles.

Hypocalcification (enamel hypoplasia) A tooth defect where the enamel is soft and undercalcified, often appearing opaque.

Impacted tooth A tooth beneath the gum tissue which is unlikely to grow out on its own because it lies against or beneath another tooth or under bone or soft tissue.

Implant A support for a crown, bridge, or denture that has been surgically placed into jawbone.

Incisors See centrals (laterals).

Inlay A solid filling that is cast to fit the missing portion of the tooth and cemented into place.

Malocclusion Incorrect position of biting or chewing surfaces of the upper and lower teeth.

Maxilla The jawbone.

Molars Teeth with a broad chewing surface for grinding food, located in the back of the mouth.

Occlusion How teeth come together.

Orthodontics Straightening or moving misaligned teeth or jaws with braces or surgery.

Palate The roof of the mouth, which is separated into hard and soft sections.

Pediatric dentistry The dental specialty devoted to the treatment of children.

Periapical The area surrounding the end of a tooth root.

Periodontics Treatment of the gums, tissue, and bone that supports the teeth.

Periodontitis Chronic inflammation and destruction of the supporting bone and tissue membrane around the roots of teeth.

Plaque A bacteria-containing substance that collects on the surface of teeth. Plaque can cause decay and gum irritation when it is not removed by daily brushing and flossing.

Post and core An anchor placed in the tooth root following a root canal to strengthen the tooth and help hold a crown (cap) in place.

Premolars Bicuspids used for grinding and chewing food.

Primary teeth (baby teeth) A child's first teeth, also known as deciduous or reborner teeth.

Pulp The blood vessels and nerve tissue inside a tooth.

Recession Gingival recession, or receding gums, which exposes the roots of the teeth.

Resin (composite) Tooth-colored filling material used primarily for front teeth. Although cosmetically superior to other materials, it is generally less durable.

Retainer A device used to stabilize teeth following orthodontic treatment.

Root canal The removal of the pulp tissue of a tooth damaged by decay or injury.

Root planing A treatment of periodontal disease that involves scraping the roots of a tooth to remove bacteria and tartar.

Sealant A thin plastic material used to cover the biting surface of a tooth to prevent tooth decay.

Secondary teeth (adult teeth) The second set of teeth, also known as permanent teeth.

Tartar Hardened dental plaque, also known as calculus.

Third molars (wisdom teeth) Molars found in the back of the mouth that usually don't erupt until late teens (if at all).

ADDITIONAL RESOURCES

ON THE INTERNET

American Academy of Pediatric Dentistry
   www.aapd.org
American Academy of Pediatrics
   www.aap.org
American Board of Pediatric Dentistry
   www.abpd.org
Children's Dental Health Project
   www.cdhp.org
National Children's Oral Health Foundation
   www.ncohf.org
Special Care Dentistry Association
   www.scdaonline.org

BOOKS
For Babies to Preschoolers

Brush, Brush, Brush! (Rookie Toddler series), by Alicia Padrón and
   Children's Press

Going to the Dentist (Usborne First Experiences), by Anne Civardi
Pony Brushes His Teeth (Hello Genius), by Michael Dahl
What to Expect When You Go to the Dentist (What to Expect Kids), by Heidi Eisenberg Murkoff

For Ages 5 to 8

ABC Dentist: Healthy Teeth from A to Z, by Harriet Ziefert
How Many Teeth? (Let's-Read-and-Find-Out series, Science 1), by Paul Showers
I Know Why I Brush My Teeth (Sam's Science), by Kate Rowan
Make Your Way for Tooth Decay (Hello Reader, level 3), by Bobbi Katz
My Tooth Is About to Fall Out (Hello Reader, level 1), by Grace Maccarone
The Tooth Book: A Guide to Healthy Teeth and Gums, by Edward Miller

For Ages 9 to 12

Throw Your Tooth on the Roof: Tooth Traditions from around the World, by Selby Beeler (author) and G. Brian Karas (illustrator)

INDEX